THE SLOW RUNNER'S NIRVANA

THE SLOW RUNNER'S NIRVANA

DISCOVERING A PATH TO JOY IN THE PRESENCE OF PAIN

CRAIG A. GROSSMAN

XEBEC
PUBLISHING

Published by Xebec Publishing, Stevenson Ranch, CA

Cover design: Paul Palmer-Edwards

ISBN (paperback): 979-8-9886493-0-4
ISBN (ebook): 979-8-9886493-1-1

Library of Congress Control Number: 2023922917

First edition

PREFACE

This book started as a sort of ethical will intended only for the very few people who matter to me or perhaps those with whom I was comfortable enough to share my beliefs or even the fact that I had beliefs. It was a very small circle, maybe six people—my wife, my children, my father, and two friends. Of those, two people read it. I was not crafting a bestseller, but sharing whatever of consequence I had learned and wished to leave behind. The stories were deeply personal, things that I had not shared with anyone. My stories were often at odds with the person I wished to be and portrayed even to those closest to me.

By outward standards, and the standards by which I had measured myself, I had what one should want—Stanford and Harvard degrees; lots of honors and gold stars for my résumé; lots of prestigious professional titles; more than enough money; more than enough material consumption; the cars I always dreamed of; the ability to dedicate myself to intellectual pursuits; the time to refine my interests and hobbies so I could hold my head high in reading, knowledge, and swagger in any of the areas of geekdom with which I identify. Somehow I snared a highly intelligent wife, and two children followed. Having pursued the twentieth-century road map to privilege and success, I had everything, but as is the cliché, so very painfully cliché, I was not happy and had learned nothing of value. So cringingly trite, but this is where I stood at the dawn of middle age.

I was a full-time father, but I had nothing important to say to my children except "Do not follow in my footsteps." My path of apparent success as a lawyer, executive, and academic was strewn with razor-sharp shards that cut deeply, were only visible to those on the path and then only when it was too late to turn back. I could only tell my children, "Do not be like me . . . ," milquetoast advice given by a father who by the very nature of the advice is a failure.

I was not happy and did not believe that happiness existed, or if it did, it was not achievable. Maybe you had to be born with some predisposition or ability I did not have. I have always been prone to depression, the clinical malady. There is a convenient excuse for failing to find contentment. My DNA makes it impossible. Whatever the cause, I never experienced joy as most people did. I was always faking it at parties, concerts, and other things that were supposed to be fun. The psychiatric class calls this anhedonia. I had no sense of contentment, just a constant awareness that life was a sentence to suffer, ending in death. Life seemed to be a curse, an unfairness imposed by parents. Procreation was the ultimate act of selfishness. The fact that half-hearted suicide attempts failed kept my joyless life and self-loathing as a flashing neon sign on every street in my life path. My continued existence was a badge of my profound failure in life.

In fact, the very first version of what would become this work was not a comprehensive philosophy as this is, nor was it a longer statement of things to leave behind with friends. It was an ethical will. It was a suicide note. I emailed it to the little group of family and friends who might have an interest in my life or death, along with a photo of me running a trail race, the Valley Crest Half Marathon in Los Angeles, generally looking like more of a badass than I really was, striding tall amid the chaparral. I asked the recipients to remember me as the guy in the photo and not the guy I was or would end up being. I did not succeed in killing myself. Life went on.

INTRODUCTION

I Am a Terrible Runner

I peaked in second grade. I got lost in my first cross-country race. I have limited knowledge, and that knowledge is limited to what I have read in books written by people with greater qualification. I'm slow, hurt, and ponderous.

This is not modesty. I am objectively bad. At my best, I shuffled out thirteen-minute miles in a marathon. My fastest half time is over ten minutes per mile, and that is over a decade in the rearview mirror. On my runs, I walk more than I run. My limitations are not subtle, as you will discover. I really do not think I am fooling anyone about my athletic prowess.

In my mind, I am a hero slaying dragons, but I know objectively what I look like on the course. A lot of people are probably thinking things that range from *Good for him for trying* to *That guy has no business being on the course.* Many probably think, *Christ, I hope I don't look that bad when I get old.* You know you look like shit during a race when the people passing you by shout, "Looking good" and "Almost there!" I hear that encouragement a lot, often at mile 8 of 26.2. No illusions. You are reading the words of a terrible runner.

I am grateful for it.

Had I been a better runner, not hurt, not diseased, running could not have held the transformative power it did for me. Running could not be the place of discovery that it has been for me if my problems were not severe and stark. Ability would mask discovery.

The true gift of this insight is that it has been alive in the present, not seen only in hindsight and nestled in regret. I know this sounds like the trite fictions coaches and managers rely upon. I'm embarrassed writing it, but it is my actual experience.

Running itself has a particular meaning in my life as it has for many others. It has been the most important thing on my path. It has kept me alive, quite literally, saving me from problems with depression and giving me a reason to continue forward.

Running had the radical power to change me precisely because I am always battling a decaying and injured body and pain, always on the edge of failure. I have an outlook and a method of seeing the world and moving through it that has brought equanimity despite what most would consider bad news and an unhappy road ahead. If I were more capable, if training were not a minefield, if finishing a race did not require me to dive down the rabbit hole with no clear way out, running could not have provided the sometimes revelatory, transformative, and always provocative experiences that it has and the learning that grew from them.

Over thousands of miles of close observation, I learned how my mind, my body, and the external world operate together. My ambitions expanded beyond the sensible limits suggested by my ability and health. I had to learn. Injuries and poor health made extraordinary demands on every aspect of training for and finishing a marathon. I was perpetually walking a tightrope. Almost any mistake was significant. Catastrophe and failure were on the menu every time I laced up my shoes. Everything mattered. I spent thousands of miles and thousands of hours in close observation and contemplation of how to move my body the required 26.2 miles in the required time. Always working and observing, testing the internal dynamic of mind and body, the external dynamic of seeing the world and acting within it. I learned.

I do live in gratitude for what I have learned and what I have experienced in the destructive testbed of the marathon. I have run with the knowledge and intent that I would be destroying myself to some extent, but I experienced extraordinary things, impossible things, moving from hobbling injury to finishing a marathon, from catastrophic physical failure to finishing. These were actual irrefutable physical experiences, not mental exercise. It was often powerful. Sometimes revelatory.

On reflection, I bring to these experiences the inquisitiveness of a scientific mind that has witnessed a miracle and demands explanation; the passion of someone who knows how to alleviate pain and do the impossible and wishes to share it with others; and the urgency of someone who hears the clock ticking loudly and wants his life to have value to others.

This is all very uncomfortable for me, entirely out of character. Accepting something as some great life truth is not in my nature. I have no faith. I do not believe or want to believe anything. The universe is too complex. There are too many factors. Claims to universal truth have always struck me as inherently flakey and almost certainly delusional. My normal outlook falls somewhere in the neighborhood of deeply ingrained pessimism, skepticism, and existentialism. So these experiences were shocking and definitely aberrant for me. I examined, repeatedly tested, and found my experience and my efforts to understand them to endure my skepticism. I ended up refining what I wished to knock down.

In the years since delivering my initial essay to family and friends, I have been forced to face my own mortality, an experience that has prompted me to share what running has taught me with anyone else who cares to know. I make no claim to sagacity. I make no claim to originality. I am sure everything I have learned was learned by others long ago and is probably expressed better, in existing philosophical and religious traditions. What I can say is that after a life of misguided learning and intellectual activity, I have come to learn some important lessons, as important as diminishing pain and moving beyond it. I have no interest in preaching, only in explaining my own experience. You can verify, discredit, or ignore my assertions as you wish.

To my mind, these lessons are too valuable to keep to myself. The crux of each story is the same—I did x and experienced debilitating pain and injury; I did y, and I traveled a very long way, relatively pain free. Ultimately, this understanding has permitted me to choose happiness.

PART I

A New Path

CHAPTER 1

An Unhappy Life inside My Head

Running grew to mean so much and ultimately birthed this book because I have a compulsive drive to learn. I always have been really good at learning in an academic sense. Learning about life, not so much.

I was great at school—Stanford and then lowering my standards to attend Harvard. Libraries have always been magical places. In college, I squirreled away books in the hidden levels, which were used primarily, according to campus lore, as peaceful places to masturbate. I was not normal enough to use the dusty rooms for that purpose. I plowed through books and built little nests where I could spend the hours. I would sneak in several feet of a turkey-and-avocado sandwich, a sports bottle filled with Old Crow whiskey sometimes with, I am ashamed to say, lemonade powder as a mixer. So provisioned, I would dive into lengthy drug-like trips, but instead of acid and a black-light poster, I had a sandwich meant for a party, disgusting alcohol, and a palace of words.

Some days I would bring a stack of books with me to the baseball stadium. You have to love a sport that you can watch while aggressively reading at the same time. Future Hall of Famer Mike Mussina may have been pitching, and my nose would be in Bentham. I still bear some pride and regularly tell my kids that in one afternoon sitting in my favorite pub, I could down a linguica-and-jalapeño pizza, a pitcher of Anchor Steam, and four books. That is an afternoon!

Law school, then highbrow legal practice, a zany ride through the internet revolution and lowbrow professoring, my entire professional existence was all about identification, digestion, and synthesis of information, then analysis of how that knowledge would apply to arcane problems like the termination of prior transfers of copyright by the descendants of the author or whether intellectual property rights could inhere in an animal. Much of what I did was such arcanum that law did not exist on the topic. I did very important work, pumping out hundred-page memoranda that cost the client hundreds of thousands of dollars and were probably never read. I did work of great social utility, rescuing characters like Lassie and Lamb Chop from decaying film libraries. While I worked in the world of entertainment, software, and media, I remained dedicated to abstract ideas.

Although I have the bulk of my ego stashed away under this ability and vocation of learning, I do not have much pride in the results. As a professional, even as a teacher and writer, my knowledge and thought meant little. Whatever I said that could have had consequence pertains to technology that is no longer relevant or issues that have long been settled by the courts.

I had one great shot to bring my legal theories into the real world via the design of a controversial search technology. It resulted in my company getting sued by every film studio, record label, publishing rights society, and others, twenty-seven plaintiffs in all. I went from general counsel of a tech venture with some Hollywood cachet to CEO of a debtor-in-possession, with my primary investors fighting each other in the boardroom as well as at home, reportedly with organized-crime goons. I ran away to a professorship more than a thousand miles from Los Angeles. Ultimately, the courts sided with the large corporations over the innovators and consumers. Shocking.

The life of the mind inside the mind for the mind does not produce a happy person. So my intellectual bent has been a handicap of sorts. I am no object of sympathy. My interests and abilities took me to good places—some wealth, some prestige, a great deal of freedom. They just kept me from enjoying any of it. At middle age, notwithstanding a life of voracious learning, I was bounded in a nutshell, and I had only bad dreams. I knew nothing of value. I had no idea how to be happy.

Running Is My Teacher

I was almost forty when I figured out I had to turn off my brain to learn anything of value.

I always eschewed the simple and the physical as pathways to any sort of understanding or even as something useful to satisfy intellectual curiosity. I have never been against physical things. My recreational and romantic interests are carnal, extreme by most standards. My sense of strength and agency during most of my life was tied to my efforts in various combat sports. Even if my efforts in wrestling, fencing, judo, karate, krav maga, etc. led to injury and humiliation, I kept throwing myself into those activities because I wanted to kick ass and think of myself as someone who could kick ass. That aggressive, oh-so-manly desire to choke out or pin an opponent or even the more fey desire to drive home a lunge with a smug *"Et la!"* as the foil triggers the buzzer are the impulses that lie behind my decision to run a marathon.

I did not start down the path to learn anything. I did it because I was unhappy with who I was and where my life had taken me. I had rejected this job and that, found myself a full-time dad, a joy but not a great CV when dudes are unzipping their professional flies to compare business achievements. I was frequently depressed, which, in turn, had major negative ramifications. I had lost a partnership in a law firm and a lovely house in San Diego and was torn from my family by a constant sense of failure. I was suicidal and had come somewhat close to closing the book. I had been in hospitals and programs, short- and long-term, residential and outpatient, helpful but not great for an ego as overblown as the one I carried as a younger man. I had much to prove to myself in the face of disappointment. I craved the physical, the carnal, the clear triumph over an opponent.

I became intimate friends with a Dominatrix who was both the cure and the cause of my continuing madness. I lived with an emotional intensity and profundity that, like a drug, made other things seem small. Every day, I faced existential questions. Every day, I was pushed ever further to the edges of physical and emotional capacity, which, in turn, magnified the daily existential crisis. Really, there were not days. I was awake for days, no day; no night; with my family; in a dungeon; on the beach, looking at pills in my hand. My life was complicated and exaggerated to an unmanageable extent. My conventional life, career, and friendships collapsed under the weight of depression and delusion.

I was also losing physical ability in yet undefined ways, so much so that I knew any attempt at a physical sport would lead to instant, significant injury. My efforts to return to the mat or gym over the prior decade had ended swiftly in minor injury, broken toes, and a bashed rotator cuff, my anger and determination always outstripping my body and ability. Eventually, I had enough sense to look elsewhere for physical challenge.

I looked to running. I would like to say something nice about my motivations here, but I cannot honestly. My life in running grew out of an unbalanced personality coupled with mental illness.

I began running, first, at the insistence of someone with the authority to insist. Running became a transformative path, and I found running fulfilling, but as a means of self-destruction. I lost almost one hundred pounds in a matter of months. I was trying to run myself out of existence. When, after so much crisis, delusion, and treatment, I started having regular glimpses into sanity and stability, running took on an entirely different, positive cast. Running was my toehold into reality and self-improvement. It was a practical thing, very much rooted in the present, physical world. It was goal oriented, and progress could be charted, demonstrated, and felt. For years, quite literally, running kept me alive. I did not work. I did not maintain any friendships or family relationships except with my wife and children. I ran. I was a dad, but it was running that kept me in the world so I could be a dad.

So I continued for years. I knew that running was the thing that stabilized, disciplined, and gave purpose and joy to my life. I knew that so long as I kept my mind churning on running and going out into the sunshine and using my body every day, I would be okay, often content, sometimes joyful. As long as I ran, there was no room for suicidal thoughts, brooding, or destructive behavior. Running was vital to me.

However, I viewed myself as just a happy enthusiast, no different from any annoying person who argues that you have not lived until you have rock climbed, skied, surfed, or skydived. I was no different. For me, the benefits were just extraordinary because my problems had been extraordinary.

A New Goal: The Marathon

After several years of finding solace on the road, I wanted more. I was never at ease being a stay-at-home dad, as it was not entirely by choice. That was always a reason to hide from colleagues, classmates, and friends. I know this is a problem of the privileged, but my friends, classmates, and colleagues were on their way to great things. Some became billionaires (that is with a *b*), ended up in the US Senate, or went on to serve as secretary of state. It seemed a given that all Stanford grads had tens of millions in the bank and were continuing on to their fourth or fifth venture as some means of self-actualization through technology development.

Meanwhile, I was at home with my kids. On substance, I won times one thousand. Being a full-time dad was incredible, but it did not support my ego and identity. I had all the titles—partner, CEO, professor, and retiring by forty—to broadcast some success, but I did not buy it. I knew the retirement was involuntary. There was always a sense of moral weakness and lack of purpose. Running was a lifeboat, but just a hobby. A hobby, by definition, is not a life.

Now, approaching fifty, I felt a sense of physical decay. The loss of my physical ability to the press of time, of years wasted, of flagging self-esteem, of a bad situation with no end. These were my motivations for announcing that I would train for a marathon. There was no *Kung Fu*–like sojourn barefoot through the desert, no David Banner (sometimes the Hulk) hitchhiking to melancholy music, just a disappointed, unfulfilled guy looking to rebuild his confidence and sense of agency.

I picked a marathon as a goal because the idea of running a marathon has cultural cachet. It is very hard to do. It is a point of pride. It would make for a cool picture in my office. That picture would be proof to me and anyone in the same room that I am formidable, that I still can kick ass in some way. I wanted to prove something to myself, affirm my worth, give the finger to the march of time and the corollary weaknesses in my body, compensate for career failures, shake my fist at the void, or something else. I set out to achieve these goals with a grim, adversarial, even violent outlook. There was nothing thoughtful or wise about it.

I may have started out to show how tough and capable I still could be, but running quickly became a point of learning and inquiry on the most important and profound topics—pain, happiness, and how to pursue the one and minimize the other. Everything of value I know arises from running. I did not start there or try to get there. My motivations were puerile and unwise, but that is the result.

Given my age and ability, I had to walk a very narrow path in training. I had to do close to everything entirely right every day to get to my goal. Mistakes were swiftly revealed and shortly thereafter punished with failure, pain, and injury, which, in turn, jeopardized the larger enterprise. In practice, doing something one way leads to pain and failure in a clear, verifiable sense. Doing that thing another way allows progress on the path toward a larger goal, on schedule and in decent health. There were not many shades of gray to ponder. There was failure and pain on the one hand, ease and meeting objective goals on the other.

In the face of failure and pain, I had to adapt and rethink. I had to learn in ways I never had before. What I know is the result of careful observation and thought over years, thousands of miles, months and months of inactivity in a boot or on crutches, and a mind running with scenarios almost all the time. Conversations and other mental activity were breaks in the stream of analysis. I extracted isolated bytes of truth, rules I could play with, validate, or destroy with an experiment. As I observed and analyzed, hour after hour poring over data collected on my runs—the objective numbers, the more subjective feelings of pain and freedom—I saw rules, shining beacons of direction. Like the laws of physics, if something is true, that truth manifests itself wherever it applies. Things never before known or understood by me were present all around me.

The learning was often uncomfortable, but I was so committed to crossing the finish line that I was willing to go through my assumptions (even things that comprised important aspects of my personality) with a scalpel, mallet, and flamethrower. A number of things hit me in the face, unexpected and unsought. My approach could mean the difference between debilitating pain and ease. In some cases, it was as extreme as smashing your hand with a hammer in one case and, in the other, not smashing your hand and then maybe even getting ice cream too. Radical results, some truly shocking and profound.

The learning did not arise from a book or reflection. It was not an intellectual exercise in finding meaning or an anxious need to increase knowledge. These were actual, largely physical experiences, moving from a world of blinding pain in one moment to continuing in the next moment and ultimately finishing.

CHAPTER 2

One Race Taught Me Most of What I Know

Revelations in the Chicago Marathon

In a prior age and different cultural context, I absolutely would have claimed that I encountered a miracle or the hand of a god or something beyond explicable existence. My experience was that shocking, that strong, that revelatory.

I do not believe in miracles. I do not believe that angels, gods, demons, aliens, chupacabras, or anything else invisible in every place except a person's head exist. Even for people who believe these things are real, there is nothing to be seen except the existence and operation of their brain. There is no reality to these things, just faith and imagination. The faith, however, is not necessarily baseless. People often say they see aliens or speak with a god to attain some kind of status in their community, even if they themselves do not hear such voices. Some people, however, do hear voices or experience what cannot be anticipated or explained. In prior centuries, these people had equal opportunity of being burned as heretics, canonized as saints, or merely assumed to have some magic or spiritual sensitivity that might qualify them to be a healer or holy person. Today, we would generally restrain these folks as unpredictable psychotics. Haldol and slippers without laces would be the modern response to people who insist they experienced something impossible or fantastic. We may pretend to believe this stuff in church, but when a guy seeing angels is dancing on our lawn, we call 911.

I heard no voices except my own authentic voice breaking through the pain. My experience, however, was definitely in the vein of a revelation, undergoing something so inexplicable and powerful that many people would look for a divine, unearthly explanation, an apparent miracle. David Hume nailed it. A claim of a miracle requires miraculous evidence. There were thousands of possible explanations for what I had seen more likely than a miracle even if I did not know them. So I do not believe I experienced an actual miracle. However, I think I do know what it feels like to experience what people experience when they insist that they experienced a miracle. The journey from debility and pain to redemption and accomplishment was that strong, that sudden, that inexplicable, that radical, that positive.

It knocked my life in a new direction and fundamentally changed my view of self and the world.

Bring It On

I finished the 2016 Los Angeles Marathon, my first, and did so no more injured than when I started. It did everything I hoped it would do for me. It provided a new idea of what I could do and who I was. I was not just a guy who had done a lot of things years ago. I was not just a runner. I could say that I ran a marathon. If I could do one more, maybe the marathon would be my distance and I could—dare I even think it—call myself a marathoner. I would not hold myself out to the world as one, because that invites the discussion I could not survive—How many marathons? What times? Inside, I was elated with my accomplishment. I was happy with myself—a rarity—and the experience was a life highlight. I was not going to stop.

I was exploring all sorts of possibilities as I continued my training.

This was my new life. I pored over every article on top-ten marathons and bucket-list races. I read hundreds of descriptions and reviews of races. I was absorbed. I assumed I would run Los Angeles again, my hometown race. It was cheap, easy, and required no extra travel or hotel. It is a marvelous ride from downtown to the sea, and maybe most important, entry was open.

Months into my training schedule, I was alerted by my credit card company about a mystery charge for a few hundred dollars for a Chicago athletic club or something like it. I explained to my bank that I was not in Chicago and could not possibly have joined a sports club or even paid for a gym pass somewhere in Chicago. I was incensed, outraged, I tell you, invaded, put upon by this fraud. I canceled the card and had a new one issued. I cursed the depravity of man; wrongly accused family members of losing or misusing the card; wondered if I had been rolled, taken to a Chicago mob front, forced to run my card, and somehow roofied into amnesia; but my wrath was misplaced. After all this wild negative imagination, I recalled that I did have a connection to Chicago. I had entered the lottery for the Chicago Marathon several months earlier. This was my entry fee. Things were breaking my way, a new, better life.

Training went well. I felt prepared. My family and I made the trip to Chicago. There I found myself surrounded by runners from all over the world, all of us en route to the race start. I felt that I was a part of something bigger than myself, as I always do in races, but particularly now among all the colors representing so many far-afield places. I shared an elevator with a team of runners from Ecuador. I could understand every eleventh word and felt very cosmopolitan as a result.

I had high confidence. I had a thoughtful plan for everything. I knew I could do it. After all, I had done it on a much harder course in Los Angeles, and my training went even better this time. Along the way, I had stumbled into the San Francisco Half Marathon with no comprehension of the hills before me, and I managed to finish that. I would be okay.

This broader confidence notwithstanding, my usual two hours of panic prior to the race—around using the bathroom and needing it again and wanting it again and again and contemplating if I could make it without using it again—began. I jumped up and down in the line for the bathroom, wondering what would make people more mad: if I pushed my way to the front or made them endure the spectacle of an older man wetting himself. Anxiety. Fear. Full bladder.

The start time finally arrived. Events overtook fear.

We were underway along the lake with the huge buildings, the architectural gems of the US on our left. Chicago is a city that looks more like a city than any other city. It is a comic-book architectural fantasy for me. The starting hullaballoo and crowds settled, lulling my high emotions into a deep, easy contentment. The buildings gave way to dappled parks and low neighborhoods. It was a good day. A great day and I knew it. This would be one of the best days of my life, but not for the reasons I assumed. It would not be the lark I thought it would be. Of course not. It would be a trial.

Pain and Failure

A marathon is accepting the thousand razor cuts of the experience. Somewhere in the race waits a mile that is a nemesis, a motherfucker born to kick you in the groin, mock your hubris for thinking you could run through her, crush your dreams, spit in your face, and laugh at your pain. For better runners, this is often mile twenty-two. For me, it came around mile sixteen, which was disconcerting because that was a comfortable training distance for me.

I started having pain in my left foot and then deep within my pelvis. Anyone who has run a race underprepared knows the feeling of the tendons stretching and giving way in the hidden structural bits we never think about, for me the pelvis and groin. Over the next several miles, the discomfort grew. It was a miserable time. My entire experience was this growing suffering. Every step hurt. I was deeply unhappy about what was happening to the race, this day, this experience into which I had invested so much work and hope and identity. My solution was to ignore it, to press on as planned, a very stupid decision.

I continued descending into the pain for maybe two miles, hobbling, my mind whirring from the growing agony and branching off to disappointment, what I had done wrong over the last six months, and many other irrelevancies.

I was splitting my time between set run and walk intervals, which I found as a beginning runner could be tweaked to get me through almost any situation. My runs turned to shuffles. I could only "run" for forty seconds instead of a minute, then twenty seconds, then ten seconds, and then my "runs" ground down to a hobble and then just a lurch forward for a few steps ending in engrossing pain and disappointment, abject despair. This sounds overblown, but this was my true state. I was caught in a swirl of torment and mental anguish. In every moment, with every impact on the pavement, every movement, I was asking myself if I could make another step, how I could go on, my mind a mélange of half-conscious recriminations about where I failed along the way—in training, in life, and in everything else leading to this disintegration of ability, of will, of hope.

On the surface, I maintained an ongoing internal monologue of what I should do next. *Okay, I'll walk for fifteen seconds, then try to run for ten seconds.* Decisions on top of decisions. *Shit. No good. No fucking good. I can't. I just can't. My quads are spasming, and I am having a hard time staying upright. Shit. Okay. Maybe if I walk for twenty seconds, I could run for eight seconds. Fuuuck. It hurts too much. Maybe if I . . . I just can't. My fucking leg won't move. Shit. No. It's no good. No good. Can't . . .* Conscious thought and reason had left as I was grinding down in spectacular failure. I was going more slowly than a walk, and every step hurt so much it was a separate act of will, each act echoed by shots of pain, and all of it laid over the systemic background torment of total depletion and fatigue.

Like a fighter at the limits of consciousness, swaying and unable to move, but with just enough muscle control to stay upright, I possessed just enough brain function to hang on to the primary desire to stand.[1]

---

1. I later learned that the physiological phenomenon of losing muscle control and brain function that I was experiencing is similar to the knockout of a boxer. I believe that I had depleted my glycogen stores, and as a result brain function began to shut down, putting my body in an immobile, unconscious recovery mode. The pain caused by my fight to remain conscious and move against my autonomic response to go unconscious defined my unhappy situation. In a boxer, I understand, each blow releases a chemical in the brain that impedes function, and with enough repeated blows, the harmful chemical is created faster than the body can eradicate it, and the brain shuts down, entering a recovery mode.

I was swaying, waiting for the final tap to the jaw that would put me to sleep.

The pain had won. I was gone. There was only the pain. My emotions and thoughts were a smeared inarticulate streak of terrible colors. I had been brought to a bedrock level of unhappiness and suffering. To the extent there was a voice, some person still inside my head, it was rapidly serving up pointless new recriminations and feelings of disappointment for the inevitable failure of the prior moment, cycles of pain to coherence and back to pain that could run several times in a second.

Objectivity Speaks

Thankfully, a different part of my mind showed up to assess the situation. A momentary shred of mental control shouted through the dross. I do not know how or why. I stopped trying to move at all. In an inexplicable window of clarity, I was able to interrupt my useless internal cycling pessimism to think as I wished to think, to be the master of my thoughts. This was a distinctly different process and a new voice in my mind.

This voice was reason, an objectivity informed by my desire and pain, but not the creature of it. Whatever internal arbiter decides these things, it gave this new voice the floor.

This new objectivity asked what I should do. There was only one decision in front of me, and it was simple: finish or quit. There was nothing else, nothing relevant, nothing to be considered, not money, not career, not the state of the world, not kids, nothing. Right then, in that place, in that moment, all there was to decide was whether I would finish or quit. Anxiety over finances, how I could duck the next PTA event, my embarrassment over farting during PE in the sixth grade (which really happened), my despair at the state of the republic, none of it mattered. I could return to all those things later, but they were entirely irrelevant now. Finish or quit? That was the only decision before me.

I examined my pain carefully, objectively, focusing on each part that hurt, to know the nature, extent, and depth of the pain. Did my pain signify that I was causing any permanent damage to myself, something that would require a sane person to quit, get treatment, and look to the next race? Did my hopes of running again require me to quit now to be able to fight (or run) another day? No. I was very familiar with the injury-like pain, both the metatarsal pain in my foot and the stretching of the tendons in my pelvis. The twitching and buckling of my thigh muscles was no mystery either. *I know what this pain is. It is an old friend, and it does not mean anything is wrong with me. Fatigue would be cured with rest. I do not need to quit for health reasons. There is no reason I should quit.*

Do I want to quit? Do I want to give up, sit on the pavement, and have the paramedics pick me up? No fucking way. Nothing can hurt enough to make me do that. I have worked too hard, dreamed of this moment in every training step for months. I have never gone five waking minutes without thinking about this day, this moment. I may have lost things in my career, health and otherwise, but this is what I have now. No, I'm not quitting. I set this as a real goal. I do not quit. They may have to peel my carcass off the pavement, but I will not quit. So I want to finish? Of course. That is why I am here and worked so hard to be here. Good. I can and will finish. Decision made. There is nothing left to be said. All that is left is getting to the finish line.

I now know what I am doing: finishing.

In every action and thought at every moment, I am doing only one thing: finishing.

That decision changed everything that day and in some ways my life that would follow.

Decision Decreases Pain!

Making the decision to finish vastly reduced my physical pain—instantly.

This is not a metaphor. It was spooky, crazy. I was still in great pain, but it was very much diminished, instantly. There was no interregnum of rest or nutrition or a comforting call with my kids. The experience was direct. Decision made. Pain reduced. Wild.

The prior indecision had infected every step and magnified every moment and every pain into something unnecessarily traumatic. *Can*

I take another step? Should I? Decisions upon agonizing decisions made on a foundation of misery and pointless looking backward to prior failures. Now, I knew what I was doing. I was finishing. I did not have to worry about anything else. Nothing else mattered. The pain was now just a nuisance to be managed, something that the overriding decision to finish placed in a different intellectual framework, and this new framework shaped my experience of the pain. It amplified or reduced it, actual physical pain, not mental anguish, not metaphorical pain, the actual subjective experience of pain in my pelvis and foot, even the systemic pain in my body. The role I gave the pain changed my subjective experience of it, radically, instantly.

The pain was still there. My body was suffering a metabolic and structural breakdown, and this hurts. If there is an objective measure of pain, the pain might be quantifiably the same, but it hurt much less and was far less important to my situation. I do not believe in miracles, but I experienced one.

Knowing What to Do Further Decreases Pain

Making the decision to finish had a significant ancillary benefit that in itself felt transformative. Once I had decided that I would finish, I knew what I needed to do. I reoriented myself to do whatever was necessary to finish. This sounds facile, even stupid, but it is profound.

Once I refocused myself on the goal, finishing, I was no longer performing or trying to live up to an expectation or desire concocted in some other world. I could now accept and deal with the present actual reality. The fantasies in my head about what this day would be and the broken dreams and disappointment that it was not so were gone as rapidly and easily as the pain was relieved. It happened with whatever minuscule electrochemical change inside my brain denotes a decision.

Having decided to finish, I could finish this race with all the conditions being as they actually were on this day. This sounds like a tautology, but it is not. Before I was wrestling with some hypothetical runner with a hypothetical body that was going to finish in such and such a time on such and such a run/walk split and have certain feelings that would make this day fantastic. All efforts on that front were useless and likely destructive because that runner did not exist. He may have existed when crushing his last training run, but he did not exist today. The conditions had changed, inside my body and on the course.

Once I understood my new goal, I had the psychological freedom to assess things as they really were. I was not going to perform as I had hoped. My prior goals were dead. I was way beyond tweaking a game plan. With the bare decision to finish no matter what, I could see the facts and obstacles as they were and do what was necessary to finish. Because I was no longer interested in a time, I walked when I wanted. I let the pain guide when I ran. I ate and drank when I wanted to or thought it wise, and my pain lessened as a result. I recovered over time. The critical meltdown passed.

I had freed myself to finish with the decision to finish.

Past Pain to Fun

An increase in certitude gave me the space to make another decision that decreased pain further and made it a better day.

I decided I should have fun. I would focus on the things around me, enjoy the city, remember the images. I made videos for my kids, sharing emotions that now ranged from serenity to outright euphoria. I was going to live this time . . . in the Chicago Marathon! It was a big deal to get to live the day I was living—after all, I had to win a lottery to get here. I was going to savor it. I was able to take my pain, already greatly reduced, and put it back, way back in my mind. I was busy doing positive, enjoyable things.

Yes, I had a lot of pain. It was there in every step, and a sane person might have quit. However, it was now just a loud background distraction that I was pushing back and back and further back. I was running the Chicago Marathon! I hurt, and on that level, things were terrible, but the pain was not what I was doing or the focus of what I was doing. It was a condition to be managed, a nagging presence. It was a barking dog next door, not in my house. Whether to let the nonstop, loud barking ruin my race or just exist as background noise was largely up to me.

Despite the pain that remained, I had a great time, a really great time. I knew this would be among the handful of days in life that I may be able to recount to my grandchildren when all other memories had faded. I knew what a gift the day was, and I gave myself permission to enjoy it.

I had enough left to run really hard in the final hundred yards. I leaped high as I crossed the finish line, perhaps a whole two feet. I had horrendous pain and almost fell upon landing, but it's a great photo.

Again, this really happened. I was stalled out with pain. I broke the cycle of my pointless thinking to assess the situation. I made a decision. As a direct result, I finished with substantially less pain, enjoyed myself, and ended up flying over the finish line. It was a remarkable experience. It was also great fun.

It is past, but I still live in gratitude for it.

PART II

How to See Clearly

CHAPTER 3

Life Is This Moment and the Next

Life itself is a series of actual moments, not ideas, plans, fears, goals, or anything else. There is nothing more, just this moment and movement to the next. Therefore, we face only two questions in life: *What is happening?* and *What should I do next?*

If we see clearly where we are and the actual, practical options for our next step, life is not complicated. Happiness requires that we step out of the fantasy and chaos in our heads to live our actual lives.

I marvel at ultradistance runners, really anyone who can do something so difficult for so long that, to me, it seems not only impossible, but terrifying to attempt. There are people who swim for twenty-four hours. How could it be possible? How could anyone run across the starting line, knowing that dozens of hours of running lie ahead, or jump into the water, knowing that they will have to survive for a day, even treading water while they eat? My awe is not limited to ultra-athletes. A trip to the corner could be equally daunting and impossible for a person of more limited physical ability. How can anyone have enough confidence to start?

I once chatted with an ultradistance runner about this. I had crossed the marathon distance barrier, but taking on one hundred miles, stringing four-plus marathons together in one day as he had done several times, just seemed impossible. When I asked this superb runner how he does it, I expected him to say something like, "It's just another distance" or "You can do it if you train properly" or "Once it is done, it is no more mysterious than a marathon, half marathon, or 10k was to you before you hit those milestones."

Instead, he shared my awe and confusion. He agreed that, looking at the task in its entirety, running one hundred miles in a day, it is impossible. No doctor would say that the human body is designed for this distance. The runner told me he could not even start if he viewed the task as running one hundred miles. He cannot think about one hundred miles or where he is on a path to one hundred miles or anything on that level.

If, this runner explained, he stopped at mile thirty, tired, maybe suffering from a blister that hurts more with each step, maybe sapped from dehydration or any of the myriad other possible failure points, and asked himself if he could run another seventy miles, the answer would always be no. He could not go on and would fail. The idea of another seventy miles is too overwhelming, and thinking about how to get through seventy miles ignores the problems at hand that are likely solvable, a sore spot, the need for carbohydrates, and so on. Instead he looks at what can and should be done at every point during the race. This limited view provides concrete questions with concrete answers and feasible actions. If, for example, he explained, he needs to stop running, the range of things to do is limited. He can eat or drink, change socks, tend to wounds, rest, or quit the race, and not much else. The one hundred miles happens, if it happens, on its own. The runner just needs to navigate the moments, making the narrow decisions and taking the few possible actions each moment presents, until the finish line appears.

In brief, the answer to the question of how someone can run one hundred miles is they cannot, nobody can. You can run through periods of time that ultimately will cover one hundred miles, but the challenge and the race take place in a series of moments. For the goal of finishing, the decision is always as simple as continuing or not continuing in each moment. You find the next metaphorical handhold and do not look down at how far you could fall or up to how much work is yet to be done. The task at mile two is the same as the task at mile eighty-two. Make decisions as they arise based on the situation as it is at that moment and the possible choices at hand. Live what is actually happening and see where it goes.

Put differently, there is no such thing as a hundred-mile run in direct human experience. "One hundred miles" is an after-the-fact description, an organizing concept for a group of related moments. In real experience, facing real problems, there are only moments and the need to address issues actually present in that moment. Working within this reality makes success possible even when all reason may point to its impossibility at the outset. The task at hand will always be manageable, making the journey plausible, one segment, one stride, one decision to the next.

This string of moments—that is your life happening. Your mind and attention can be elsewhere. You can build castles of fear and worry in fantasy, but these moments, each step, each moment—that is your real life whether your mind is there or elsewhere.

The Moment Is Simple

Life is simple. We stand in a solitary moment. We have to decide what to do to shape our path to the next moment. We may yearn for complexity, but this is all we have. Reality has baked into it therefore a simple paradigm for living. We always and only need to answer

What is happening now?
What should I do next?

That is our situation now. That is it tomorrow, Saint Crispin's Day, and every second until the clock runs out on our quantum plane. There is not more. This is the complete nature and run of our lives.

We make life unnecessarily complex and frequently unmanageable by avoiding this simple paradigm—What is happening? What should I do next?—and opting instead to dwell in internal worlds of our own making, demanding to know what cannot be known or do what cannot be done.

The question "What is actually happening now?" is objective, concrete, answerable. It leaves no room for scenarios based on fears, fantasies, or even hypotheticals. It requires observation, not conjecture. What is happening is usually simple, even if hard to discern. The moment may look small. It tends toward the basic and simplistic because that is our normal circumstance: simple.

What is actually happening in this instance in the real world for me, not stuff solely inside my head as I write? A good answer for me would be "I am sitting at my computer, typing," not "I am writing a book," and definitely not working to leave something behind for my children or regain lost purpose. Long-term goals and ambitions should guide decisions, but the decisions themselves are made in specific points in time, and in each moment, it is a small, manageable universe of things actually happening.

Knowing what is happening makes answering the question "What should I do next?" possible and tractable. The range of possibilities in each moment is limited, and those possibilities are usually much simpler than we would like to believe. If the possible answers to "What should I do next?" are too numerous and complex to juggle, you probably are not framing the question of "What is happening now?" properly.

Most things are binary choices. Go or stop. Life itself, like a run, is usually a black-and-white choice—finish or quit, continue with the task or do something else. In most cases, there really is not much of a choice. Almost always, there is a clear path in front of us. We may not want to follow it, but if we know where we would like to go, the best option is usually clear.

This paradigm—What is happening now? What should I do next?—is the lab experiment that is our life. There is a changing environment, things happening around us, not just inside our heads, and we make decisions in response.

That is our real life happening, now and . . . now.

Fantasy Is Complex

Sports offer clean metaphors—a defined playing field, unchanging rules, clear goals, and an emotional association with achievement and victory. A hitter only faces one pitch at a time. His decision is to swing or not swing. My impulse is to say that my life and everything around it are not so simple.

I look at myself and see an ineffably complex, even grandiose being in such large, important situations, so difficult I pay a professional to listen to me talk about them. I have issues with relationships great and small that reach into the lives of other people, a lifetime of dreams and aspirations informed by literature and culture, nurtured and thwarted, dreams of who I hoped I would be and the reality of who I am; illness, mortality, and pain; the anxiety of my children's problems; and my own wrenching feelings over the suffering in the world. I have been atop the dais, receiving an award, and a certified mad man, brooding at night with pills in my hand, checking into places where they do not let you have pills in your hand (instead they come in a tiny paper cup). Really, my situation is so out of hand I should pay someone to guide me through fifth-grade-ish craft projects (now called art therapy) just to detox and escape from the complexity. It is all so interesting I should write about it and tell everyone. Clients, family, the world . . . Could my situation possibly be as simple as the batter's asking only if he should swing? It is.

The place where we think, work, and hopefully find contentment, the place where we actually lace up our shoes, put our fingers on the keyboard, get on the train to work, play with our kids, and move is a much smaller and simpler thing than we may think or want it to be. It is a real, objective, shared reality, a world outside our heads.

However big, complex, and challenging things seem, there is no escape from the truth written in the nature of time itself. Your existence as an actor strutting and fretting on life's stage is this moment and what it holds—you and a decision about what to do next. Trying to go beyond the decision and pathways at hand is usually misguided and will misguide. The expanded scope of concern itself may make possible things impossible.

We may want life to be more complex to add interest to our situation and expand our role as an actor in the drama we concoct. We may want to see deeply into the future. We may want to correct errors or battle demons of our past. We may want to carry our present moods and aspirations into the moment, but these things are beyond our knowing or do not exist outside our mind. They are primarily fantasies, stories we like to tell ourselves. We live in a real moment, this moment, right now moving into right now.

Siddhartha Gautama, aka the Buddha, put it succinctly in the oft-attributed quote "Do not dwell in the past, do not dream of the future, concentrate the mind on the present moment."

The Rewards of the Moment

You may want to view your life as more than *Now I am running, now I am sitting on the toilet, now I am working.* It seems bleak to ditch the stuff in church about us being quasi-divine embodied angels or the stuff in the movies about us being heroes imposing justice on a disordered universe. However, keeping attention on what is really happening and what can be done in the moment does not shrink your world. By keeping the mind in the moment, we reclaim the moment. We get that moment as a piece of our lives.

Most of the time, we are on autopilot. We move, do habitual things like eat and drink, drive to and from work often in a half-aware state. We carry on conversations with words flowing without thought, spewing canned scripts. We may not be zombies. We may be highly aware, but our attention is on something not immediately present.

If you are eating cereal over the sink while you replay some hurtful thing that happened at work, chastising yourself for things you could have said, or even just fiddling with your phone or watching television, you are missing the experience of eating. Your mind is elsewhere, somewhere other than your objective life. You do not taste the food, really. You certainly do not appreciate the sensory experience of eating—the taste, smell, feel, and deep carnal pleasure of satisfying a need—that is a universe in itself.

There are worlds on end in the moment. That is your life, and it is as compelling as any fiction.

Living the simple moment to moment to moment in addition to reclaiming the moment and the next that comprise our lives has a wonderful side benefit—the potential for immediate happiness.

One finding in the new field of happiness studies is that being in a state of "flow"—completely engaged in a task, unaware of time passing, not considering anything else except the task—is critical to being happy. We need to live in the world actively, rapt, fully focused to find happiness. To be happy, we have to leave the hypothetical conversations in our mind, rehashing memories, regurgitating emotions from prior, usually negative, experiences. We have to put our creative, imaginative powers in service of our chosen path, not lose ourselves within them. We are happy when mind, body, and environment have merged, and that demands the abandonment of all but the rolling present.

At various times in life, I could sleep only after dining on the psychiatric pharmacopoeia, large doses of sedating drugs, not for pleasure or real relaxation, but simply to turn off the noise. This is hardly a complete solution. Anesthetized is not the same thing as serene. It is pumping out water from the hold of a ship that has a gaping hole in its hull. The monster, the active mind always churning and branching off into endlessly refined pathways, is merely asleep, but it is waiting to rise.

Running has been an important solution for me here, but it could have just as easily been sewing or vacuuming or tap-dancing or any other engrossing activity that relaxes the mind even in its most agitated state. Running literally placed me into the world, getting me to a starting point and digging a claw into reality. Running invests the mind and body in real, practical problems that demand solutions, not excuses, right now.

Those with the attention and discipline to live the moment unguarded will be happy. The rest of us must carve out time for some activity that forces us into the moment, into life. To the extent I was running, I was living my actual life, not the dark fantasies and intellectual diversions of my mind. Even though I am a failure as a runner and successful as an intellectual by outside metrics, running was the vocation that joined me to the world.

The Costs of Rejecting the Moment

There is a cost to bucking the paradigm of now moving to a new now. Looking beyond the things actually present in a moment misdirects us and may make good decisions impossible. If the broad fears, insecurities, expectations, and all the other things on which we ruminate are present in a moment, knowing what to do next is impossible. We are putting things in the moment that are not there, and as a result our decisions and actions may be responses to phantasms in pursuit of chimeras.

Bringing Things into the Moment That Are Not There

Bringing things into the moment that are not there exchanges real life for a purely internal game. Ultimately, fantasy crashes against reality. If during a training run, for example, the knot in my Achilles tendon is hurting in a way that I know signals further running will deepen the injury, my sole focus should be how to handle the actual situation. What to do next is a nonchoice: quit for now.

Yet even with only one real option, only one sane thing to do, I often choose insanity. I compound the problem by continuing to run, maybe even running harder as I conflate success with the endurance of pain. When I acted, I knew objectively that I was harming myself and moving away from a life-defining objective, but in that moment, I was addressing more pressing, emotional problems. The injury was making me feel keenly helpless, old, weak, all of it tied into other failures and self-loathing. Quitting, the sane, practical choice, only gives credence to these doubts and fears. So against all sense, I run. I run hard. I pick a road sign, and I sprint to it through the pain to prove to myself that I am strong and will succeed. Stupid. I know I am being stupid. My daughter has just given me her standard advice, "Daddy, don't be stupid," and there I am making a disastrous decision to satisfy a transitory emotional need. It is delusional, literally, putting imaginary things into the present reality, and it is temporary. I act based on what feels good in the instant rather than what is actually a wise, productive thing to do. I am left in a boot for months and suffer the emotional blow and financial cost of not making the event for which I was training.

If I had not conjured so many imaginary enemies and psychological needs into the situation, if I had just limited my scope to what was actually happening, namely Achilles pain on a training run that signals injury, I would not have even been tempted to do something so injurious and off the mark in terms of solving my actual immediate problem. If I had kept my focus on the moment as Mr. Gautama advises, I would have understood my options were continue or quit, and between those two, quitting is the only sane choice.

Trying to Do Things That Cannot Be Done

It is also easy to go off track with equally painful consequences by seeking to do something that in the practical living of one moment to the next, cannot be done. The folly that kept me pinned to failure in Chicago was not understanding this. The thing I was trying to do, run a marathon with a certain physical and emotional content, was not something that could be done. Having a great marathon day was too large, a broad organizing idea or description of a result, not a specific action I could take in the face of a breakdown on the course.

I was not the runner I thought I was or wanted to be. The world was not as I thought it would be or wished it would be. Things were unfolding in unanticipated, generally terrible ways outside my planning and expectations. To finish, I had to jettison all useless ideas and emotions. I had to change the scope of my view to the present, what was really happening and what I could do. When I looked at what was happening (on a street in Chicago, hanging on to consciousness, pain in the groin, unable to move after eighteen miles, injury, and nutrition problems), where I wanted to go (the finish, another eight miles), and what action I could take in the moment (rest, water, food, quit)—when I embraced the reality of the moment—the next steps were clear among the few options (rest, move, or quit). I finished.

A Broader View May Ensure Failure

If the frame of reference at the outset is too broad, you may be ensuring failure before starting.

The answer to whether you should try to run one hundred miles is almost certainly no before you take a single step. Viewed as a whole, it is an impossible task likely to end in injury. The frame of reference is too large. The same is true if during the race the runner asks himself, bloodied and tired at mile thirty, if he should go another seventy. The answer is no. The only conclusion and sane choice is to quit, maybe try again later, but quit now.

The race will end in failure even if the complications discussed above—fear of failure, anxiety over what one's pain level will be in ten miles, backward-looking frustration over mistakes that led to the present problems, and other negative emotions—do not mischaracterize the picture. If the question is "Continue running one hundred miles or quit?" there is always a clear rational choice: quit. The inquiry itself assures failure. That was my situation in Chicago. If I framed the question before me as whether I could run the marathon and have the grand day in my fantasy, the answer was no, and I would have denied myself the chance at finishing. If the question is what to do right now—run, rest, or quit—I can continue and finish.

The difference between success and failure can be how broadly to frame the inquiry. Viewed as a whole, running one hundred miles is somewhere between very unwise and impossible, yet each moment may be manageable.

Viewed broadly, everything that the runner can do in a moment is a Band-Aid to stanch a hemorrhage. However, in the moment, it is extremely helpful and may be more and more important to the endeavor over time. It is unfair to hold up the benefit of taking some water next to the overall task of running one hundred miles or even a half marathon. A fairer comparison would be the cumulative positive effects of all positive measures that can be taken over the course of the race, and that is complex and unknowable. The only thing to do is keep one's mind on the moment and navigate that moment to the next.

A small decision in a moment is much easier to make than a grand definitive decision relating to something large: a career, a project, or life itself. Quit or run for the next five seconds is an easy choice. Terminating a three-year-long, engrossing project is a heavy thing to contemplate. As with the runner, making those serial simple decisions may take you farther than you would have thought possible.

Thinking Ahead Is Impossible

A practical reason for keeping the inquiry narrow is it is simply impossible to know the future or even game out possibilities.

Much of our anger or worry over choices comes from thinking too far ahead. We can only go left now, and we worry if there is another yet-unknown opportunity to go right in the future. Once a decision gets tied up in more than one or two possibilities that may follow, the decision at hand becomes impossible. There are simply too many possibilities, and the outcome is, at that point, almost certainly far beyond our prediction and control. Even if each decision point has just two possibilities—say, continue or quit—thinking three choices ahead requires juggling eight possible combinations of decisions in one's mind. If each step has three possibilities, your universe of possible paths mushrooms to twenty-seven. We are then paralyzed because we do not know what to do and because whatever we do, the outcome is beyond our control, the choices incomprehensible in their number and permutations and still probably not even the actual choices we will face in the future. Our overly large scope leads only to anxiety over the unknowable.

Most people have been asked the classic job interview chestnut "Where do you want to be in five years?" The answer speaks to one's ambitions, but for whom has it been an accurate prediction of where one will go? The truth is most of us will have multiple careers and even more jobs; get and lose a spouse; be hit with unforeseen illnesses, gains, or losses; make choices with unintended consequences; and so on. I went to Memphis, Tennessee, to teach with the thought of staying two or three years until the next teaching gig. I am from and love my native Los Angeles. I worked in the entertainment and software arenas. I had never set foot in Memphis. If you had told me at any point prior in my life that I would leave Los Angeles to move to the South and would have a family and raise children there, I would have laughed. Objectively, the odds would be many, many thousands to one against it, but so it was. Every occurrence is such an improbable outcome, but there has to be some outcome. The impossibly unlikely is what we live every moment.

We can only observe and make the best decision possible at the time. That is truly all there is: the moment.

Why Do We Want to Be Anywhere but Where We Are?

The interesting question is not why we would choose to operate in a small, immediate real world. What is puzzling is why do we want to live a difficult pretend life as our real, simple life goes by disregarded? This is perverse and puzzling, especially when one considers that the world inside our minds often is not a pleasant place to be and the real world offers real treasures and fulfillment.

I encourage you to observe the stream of consciousness inside your own mind. You cannot in the moment appreciate what is happening, as the mind jumping from image to memory to feeling to who knows where is an involuntary experience. It is a waking dream. When you snap out of it, however, you can retain a fleeting memory of the useless journey your mind has taken. You will see that your mind is not the ordered place attached to reality you may think it is. As you sit in the car, your mind may wander to the song on the radio, then your association of the song with a girl and a scene in high school, then to what you need to pick up on the way home, then to your anger at the price of a thing, and then back to driving, all in a matter of a few seconds. With practice, at least post hoc, you can observe your mind and hopefully turn it into an ally or at least be present as a director of the films vying for attention within your mind.

This takes a great deal of practice to achieve. The typical path from an uncontrolled mind swimming in its own sea of memories and biases to a directed mind seeing and reacting to reality in furtherance of goals is disciplined meditation of some form, but why? Why is it so difficult for us to see simple reality, the place where our lives are passing us by largely unnoticed? We want our lives to be vastly more difficult than they typically are. If they are not, we want to look at something else to hold our attention.

Simply staying in a moment in reality is uncomfortable for many. We want distraction no matter how fabulous and interesting the real world around us might be. I regularly see people on a ride at Disneyland (not in line, but in a boat on Pirates of the Caribbean or another ride), looking at their phones. I regularly see people at tables in Vegas, looking at their phones. I think if someone could simultaneously ride a roller coaster, draw a natural blackjack, and have their fantasy man/woman/x underneath the table, they would be looking at their phone.

The drive to diversion is greater than a desire to skip through the bad and boring bits of life. We cannot tolerate being present in our own vacations.

Perhaps we are victims of our own cognitive ability. We have fantastically capable brains. We can create hypothetical scenarios and test them in our minds, thinking in abstractions and symbols. We can regurgitate the past and conduct mental experiments to see if things would have turned out differently if we had acted differently. These marvelous tools powered our climb up the food chain, but applied to our everyday existence, they add fictive difficulty to our situation. If we cannot find sufficient complexity in our own situation to satiate the brain, we distract ourselves with something else. It seems our brains are always looking for something more than or different from the things the simple reality of the moment can offer.

For most of us in first-world wealth, our lives are primarily a cushy exercise in eating, sleeping, defecating, and taking care of and cleaning up after the foregoing, all bookended by decades of relative helplessness. Your dog may not be able to add or even consider that eating x made him vomit last time, so maybe she will not eat something with the same characteristics as x today. However, your dog and you face the same fundamental questions every second. What is happening right now? What should I do next as a result? The fact that your dog does not castigate himself over prior mistakes or worry about scary potential futures lying at the end of a bunch of "what if" hypotheticals may be why your dog always seems more content than you are.

We usually do not have to observe, analyze, and react. Our minds may have the potential power and speed of a Saturn V rocket, but most of the time we are going from the couch to the fridge, shoving food in our gob, relieving ourselves, and repeating that cycle. Perhaps our challenge is to follow the lead of our dog more of the time.

Rejecting the Life of the Mind for the Mind

A lot of people, like me, tend to view the movie in our minds—not what is happening on the street outside the theater—as reality. Our consciousness, energy, and concern are dedicated to building and tearing down things inside our head, both the building and tearing down being entirely mental creations. To me, life is usually at its most complex and uncontrollably burdensome when I am sitting still, alone, without distraction. We may deny our devotion to some imaginary realm, but watch your brain. Much of your life is spent in a purely internal drama. Why?

I and my kindred anxious worriers like living or at least have been habituated to living in this intellectual, internal fugue. School, peers, and lots of other things surrounding us reward this bent. You can get praise for it, get paid for it. I used to get good money to write down every conceivable risk and possibility for clients or to plot the best possible path for a business with chandeliers of contingencies diverting from it, memos and contracts measured in hundreds of pages. The work product would not help anyone reach a practical decision, but that was not my job. My job was to worry and obsess over someone else's possible problems better than they could.[2] Viewed positively, this is called thinking and is often even confused with wisdom. My real-world professional, ego, and economic interests all supported a retreat into a world of mental creations. The fantasy world in my mind defined my place in the real world. To look outside my mind at what I was doing in objective, real-world terms would be a threat to my personal and social identity, my self.

Perhaps some people can create and live within a purely mental architecture that is superior to reality. If you created an internal life dedicated to your own sybaritic pleasure and had other people seeing to every real-world need, I would have a tough time demonstrating that the world outside the theater is better than the movie you are writing

---

2.   My work as a highbrow lawyer often had no practical purpose other than to provide cover to the person commissioning the work. If anyone asked the corporate officer or whomever else whether everything was given sufficient consideration, they could point to the tomes of research and analysis I produced. The huge lawyer bills would only bolster the case of the officer that he really did all he could to consider all possible liabilities and options. As such, the research and analysis were useless. The point of the exercise was to create a pile of paper and huge bills. The content, what I was actually paid to do, was largely irrelevant.

and directing in your mind, particularly given the level of misery in the real world. The debate there is the classic reality versus the lotus eaters (happy drug users) in Greco-Roman mythology or the virtue of being a childlike person versus an observant person in some Buddhist traditions. In terms people in Los Angeles would understand, it would be choosing the blue pill that offers fantastic pleasures pumped into their brain in the Matrix and eschewing the red pill and reality.

For people like me, there is not a reality versus fantasy debate to be had, because the internal, self-created world is not one that makes us happy. We use it as a means of pointless self-torment, worrying without purpose. Unless you are in this purely hypothetical, as of now impossible, class of people who can live entirely within their minds happily and without consequence, life inside the mind is not a strategy for happiness.

Working in abstraction and having one's real-world identity springing from that work does not have the feel of a tragedy. However, the more time you spend inside your head, the harder it is to leave. Worse yet, like a horror or sci-fi movie of nested dreams inside dreams, it may become impossible to distinguish real from imagined elements in your experience.

You may want to say, "This is not me. This is the life of the insane mind." Yet science has shown to an effective certitude much of what you remember clearly as critical components of your life story never happened. The neural network in your head is a scoop of potato salad composed of overlapping and blended elements of experience, including the fictions you consumed and concocted. The sane person's insanity may be never figuring out that the email or book never said what they think it said, that what they remember never happened, and that they never surface enough to distinguish what is from what they know.

Happy or not, a life inside the mind cannot help you reach the places you wish to go, because you are busy chasing chimeras inside your skull. As such, it cannot increase the contentment, sense of self, and even joy that flow from working toward and maybe reaching real-world goals. It is a distraction at best and often harmful. To be happy with an internal mental life requires a total detachment between reality and personal fulfillment, and that is delusional insanity.

To reach a real goal, our mind must be put in service of that goal. We must look at what is actually happening and decide what we can do to advance toward that goal. Any consideration beyond this and you are pursuing a different goal. Most likely, you are going nowhere.

Without any set intention, we are driven by our mental whims, not toward our desired destination. We drift in and out of our mind, jumping from one line of thought to another, jumping from one memory to another, without any reason or even awareness that we are entering into thought or changing one thought for another. We are lost and usually not even aware that we are traveling.

The mind is a powerful tool. We are smart. We are creative. That does not make us wise or happy. Happiness requires living our actual lives.

Get out of your head. Live your actual life.

CHAPTER 4

Seeing Clearly

Seeing what is happening is the essential challenge in life.

Seeing clearly demands a constant fight against concepts, language, and other biases.

Seeing clearly what is happening demands a ruthless drive to accept new facts and reject things that are no longer true, no matter how one cherishes the incorrect beliefs.

Seeing clearly demands a destruction of self. A static idea of who you are is a distorting filter that makes seeing things clearly impossible.

Dramatic fiction and our interpretation of human events usually rest on the difficulty of making a high-stakes decision, acting in the face of adversity, or both. "Mr. President, I must have the launch codes," or "Should I give up my job as a news executive to be with her?" Some stories tease out the emotions around actions, such as pursuing a dream, fighting for justice, or persevering through the storm. Many stories do both, arguing over life-and-death decisions as the protagonists struggle to survive in the snow after the plane crash.

In fact, it is often said there are only a few stories to be told: person versus person; person versus self; person versus fate; person versus nature; person versus society; person versus the unknown; and person versus technology. So which of these paradigms feature the salient act where the person observes and understands what is actually happening?

None. The need and difficulty of understanding the situation is not consciously present. The situation is a given. This moves the story along but pulls it further away from real life.

In reality, understanding what is happening is a profound personal challenge, making decisions and acting less so. It requires being clear-eyed and honest in assessing every situation. Seeing the world as it is also means retaining the flexibility to adapt to new facts and change one's assessment of what is happening as new information arrives, without any attachment to the prior view.

If you wish to live in the real world, not in a world of fantasy and emotions, you must see what is happening.

Seeing Clearly Is a Life Discipline

Seeing the world as it is requires us to stretch our relationship with the world as much as we can toward objectivity, to transcend our place in the world. The Buddha said it succinctly: "We make the world with our minds." In a very real sense, certainly real to you, the world exists because your eyes see, your ears hear, and so on. The world is something you have made in your mind. The philosopher Alan Watts puts it more poetically. To him, your eyes evoke the stars; your ears evoke the sound of the tree falling because without eyes to see, there really is no such thing as starlight or even light; and without ears there is no sound. One can argue with the language, but the crux of the point is unassailable. We, these beings with eyes and ears and brains, have a great deal to do with how the world exists because the sound of the falling tree exists only in our heads, and sight of the tree exists only in our heads. That is our predicament as humans. To the extent possible, we must see without ourselves, yet the world exists subjectively only as a thing we sense and try to make sense of. The task is logically impossible, but we must strive to see the objective world we share with others if we are to live happily in it.

It is work. To know what is happening you have to look with intention. You have to see what is happening. You have to pay attention and catalog what you see. This sounds too obvious to state and too easy to worry about, but most of us participate in the world we inhabit without paying any attention to it. While our eyes are physically open, the images somehow flow through us like background noise to our running thoughts. We are pushed and pulled by circumstances. Instead, we need to take the position of a curious, outside observer to see what is happening. This is not intuitive, but it can be learned and trained. The benefits of doing so, of paying attention to the world in which we operate, are huge in terms of moving through it productively, but also in moving happily. Stress, confusion, and many other problems lift when attention is brought to what is happening in the moment.

Careful, real-time observation is a different way of seeing, of thinking, of living. It also carries an immense gift—a world that is endlessly interesting and often beautiful.

This is not easy. It is a discipline.

Organizing Concepts and Words Change What We See

To navigate the world, we rely on concepts of what things are, how they behave, and how they are relevant to us. The words we have are closely linked to this model of the world we are always building in our head. If you know the word, you know the concept or behavior. If there is no word for something, you probably cannot see it. We need to recognize immediately that the thing coming toward us is a car, the shapes under our feet are stairs, and the thing next to us is a person, a special person, our spouse. Car, stairs, and spouse are ideas and broad descriptions of what is seen, however useful they may be. They are not what we see, and we must see facts shorn of organizing concepts and conclusions. To do otherwise is to skirt reality, limiting what you see to things within concepts and conclusions or possibly limiting what we see to realms of fantasy inside our head.

It is another great conundrum. To see what is actually happening, we must see the world without concepts and words, and yet we need concepts and words to help us make sense of what we see. We must try to see what everything in our experience trains us not to see. This requires constant attention and adjustment.

The big point is to see that what we think we see is not necessarily what is. We are trapped, looking at the world through the mail-order X-ray specs of language and the culture that birthed it. I am not saying it is even possible to escape these distorting forces entirely, nor am I saying that words and concepts are bad. They are essential. Without them we are totally at sea, unable to understand and act. The great challenge is to see the external world as clearly as one can, using words and concepts to understand what one sees and not to let words and concepts distort what one sees and to be on guard for those lurking distortions.

There are a number of ways our operating concepts and words distort what we see.

Concepts Lead Us to Misinterpret What We See

I grew up and now live in a desert. As a kid, every group hike and school trip was preceded by a talk about snake safety. The adults carried snakebite kits with razors (not a good thing). I am terrified of snakes all the time. I am always on the lookout when running. Frequently, I see a snake, switch into a fight-or-flight mode, and run out of the way in a broad arc, estimating the length of the radius and trying to remember how far a rattler can jump.

When I get close enough, any confusion melts, and it invariably turns out to be a piece of a tree, part of a bike tire, anything but a snake. Now I see the object differently, for what it is, and I can no longer see a snake when I look at it. Now I can only see a plastic bag or whatever it really is. Before, I really saw a snake. I was not wondering if that ambiguous thing ahead could be a snake. I saw a snake. My heart raced. I saw a snake! With the concept of snake firmly planted in my awareness, my mind forced ambiguous facts to fit the concept.[3]

In my strangest snake run-in, I am jamming along a sandy creek (because in Southern California, rivers have no water), feeling a very spry and nimble thirty-nine at the time. Far ahead of me I see a large, long branch lying across the width of the trail. The branch is big enough that I plan my steps so I can leap over it. Only when I was in the air above it and looked down did I see the branch was a large rattlesnake stretched to its full, terrifying length. I did not think it was a snake or possibly could be a snake until I was literally over it and looking at the scaly pattern on its back. What I saw did not fit my concept of what a snake on a trail would look like. I have since learned that a great number of people pick up snakes, believing they are sticks. Surely, when they looked at the object, they saw a stick and had no doubt that they were reaching for a stick and not something ambiguous that could also be a snake. I am not alone.

I experience an even more bizarre example of the mind replacing reality with a concept of what the reality is. I have audio pareidolia. This means I hear things that are not there. More specifically, I misinterpret sounds that are there. The phenomenon is much the same as seeing animals in clouds except you are certain the animals are real. It is not uncommon or dangerous, but it is instructive. I hear the faint sound of a radio or television on in another room. It usually sounds like something odd like military band music or an old-timey blow-by-blow

---

3.   As with so much else I have written, I later learned that other, wiser people have come to the same conclusions sometimes thousands of years before I did. In fact, I learned the snake example is an allegory in Buddhism and other Indian traditions. Perhaps there is something hardwired in our brains to see snakes in every squiggle. This is deflating, like working for years to invent something and then learning you can buy a better one at Home Depot. It is also validating. I am very confident that what I say has merit and is likely correct. Wiser people have reached the same conclusion and written about it, and millions of followers have found their conclusions to be true. All I can bring to the dance is my independent discovery of these ideas in my own twenty-first-century experience. I am sure in many places what I write conflicts with established philosophical traditions. Press on those points extra hard to see if they are solid.

call of a boxing match in fast-talking 1930s style. I know what I am hearing is impossible. I know there is no device that could be on, but there it is, the ragtime jazz or 1945 football commentary or whatever. I have been down this path before. I know this is not happening, a trick of the ear, and I try to ignore it, but I cannot unhear the music or voices or whatever it is. Hours may pass, and even though this misapprehension happens, I know this misapprehension happens, and (here is the kicker) what I am apprehending is in fact impossible, eventually, I am certain this time something is on. I hear it. I walk from room to room. I may end up crawling under tables. Ultimately, knowing my history, I try clicking noise sources on and off. The music or voices I heard so clearly and could not unhear despite my logical arguments against it turn out to be the hum of a fan or clothes dryer or something like it. It is unsettling.

It seems we often begin with a working concept of what something is when we apprehend it. Then we see only the thing defined by the concept and cannot see it otherwise. Uncertainty is difficult to find, as we can see things through the lens of only one concept at a time. If you look at a classic optical illusion, you can see two faces or the candlestick defined by the contours of the faces. You can cycle back and forth between seeing a candlestick and seeing faces, but you cannot see both faces and the candlestick at the same time, nor can you not see the faces or candlestick once you have found them in the image. You can only see faces or a candlestick, not both, not neither, but either one or the other.

Concepts Shape How We See Things

Even when we are looking at a thing and know it is the thing we see, concepts still shape what we see. Perhaps the more intimate a concept is, the more it shapes perceptions. My youngest child started driving. I look at them, so small in the seat, the little face of an eleven-year-old peering over the wheel, and it seems absurd that this baby is driving. Yet objectively, they are sixteen. They are not small. They are average height. They look completely appropriate for their age. My concept of them determines what I see. You would see them as a sixteen-year-old learning to drive, not I. The same is true of my older child. She is a young woman, actually above average size, mature beyond her years. Yet I look at pictures of her in her lab coat and think it is so cute that she is dressed up like a scientist as if she were going to fourth-grade career day and not fiddling with Ebola in a real bio lab. If my younger one registers at about eleven years of age, she will perpetually look about fourteen to me. Here, I do not see or hear things that are not there as in the snake and radio examples, but my concept of who my children are, how they actually exist and fit in my life, shades my interpretation of what I see.

Continuing with the concept of a person shaping the way a person is seen, I do not recognize myself in photographs. I do not think I live in vanity-driven denial. I have very little hair on top of my head. When I look in the mirror, I see myself. I do not see an Adonis with flowing locks. If you asked me to provide an objective description of how much hair I have, I could do so accurately. Yet many times I am looking at a photo and wondering who the bald guy is. After a couple of seconds of examination, I see that this guy is wearing my shirt, sitting right where I was . . . That guy is me. I am surprised. In the photograph, I look more like my grandfather than the way I look to myself in the mirror. It is like hearing a recording of your voice and having to confront the fact that yes, you do sound like that. When I look at myself in the mirror, I simply do not see the same thing as I do when I look at myself in a photograph without knowing the person is me. The dimensions and color, all the objective things, are the same, but the images register as very different things because I am beginning with a different set of expectations.

Concepts Can Replace Reality Altogether

Beyond shaping what we see subtly (I know I am bald, but I do not look like a bald guy) and misapprehending what is actually there (what are the best boots to keep a stick from biting your leg), it is easy enough to observe with absolute moral certainty things that were never there. A skilled lawyer can get people to see whatever he wants them to see. A dozen sober people on a jury can watch the same video. After getting a bunch of softball questions—"Did you see the man in the blue baseball hat?" Yes. "Did you see him cross the street?" Yes. "Did he cross from the top of the screen to the bottom, that direction?" Yes. "Did he cross before or after the yellow car went through the intersection?"—now there is disagreement. The jury breaks into opposing camps—those who say yes and those who say no, some unsure, some professing it was clear as day. There may be yelling and aspersions cast on the intelligence and vision of the jurors with differing memories when, in fact, there was no yellow car. The question proffered by an authority with knowledge implied the existence of a yellow car and therefore changed the memory of jurors to include a yellow car.

It is established beyond doubt that eyewitness testimony is extremely unreliable to the point of being meaningless or misleading in many cases. On probative versus prejudicial value, eyewitness testimony is probably the least reliable form of evidence and something so regularly flawed it would not be regarded as useful in many cases if we did not have a cultural tie to the notion that "seeing with your own eyes" makes something real. Real money, guns, bodies, documents, etc. state unequivocally what they are without any filter of concept or failure of memory. Witnesses and jurors are piles of ego and bias just waiting for the right question to catalyze fantasies into professions of truth.

I could go on with more examples. The phenomenon is everywhere. We do not see what is there. We do not see the information our eyes take in. We see what we think we see, and that is the function of the conventional model of the world we have built in our heads, the world described by the language and culture we have. That, however, is not the world. We need to see the world. That is where we live. That is our challenge.

The Problem of Letting an Authority See for You

The medical profession frequently falls victim to its military-like hierarchy, a hierarchy resting on the assumption that the person with more stripes on their arm always knows better. As a practical and definitional matter, the senior doctor is always right because she gets to determine what is right and write it in the chart to make it official. But the stripes and the desire to believe that authority tracks competence gets in the way, burning a governing concept into the process that trumps all observation and data. Doctors opt for blindness and often reject what is plainly visible because the writing in the chart demands it. The hierarchy demands it.

Early in the process of a decade-plus-long journey of seeking a diagnosis, I had a brain MRI. The anonymous doctor behind the curtain of medical imagery said it showed an infarct. I played the MRI frame by frame forward and backward trying to see what the radiologist saw. I could not, but I am a mere layman. I should hardly even be allowed to look at these images. If the radiologist says x is here on this frame, my not seeing x hardly signifies. I had to defer to the vastly superior knowledge and authority of whoever read and reported on the images. My treatment went forward with local neurologists and other doctors. Things did not improve, and all the while I was aware of the risk of a bigger, more destructive bleeding on the brain. The belief that I had a small stroke and that a larger one would be coming and things were not getting better was stress on stress. Fortunately, I was helping a brilliant professor of anesthesiology bring his invention to market. He was kind enough to get me royal treatment at a first-rate medical research center. I saw their grand old man of ophthalmology. He was as senior and as accomplished in his field as one can hope to be, full professor, head of his group in the hospital, and respected researcher. In his world, he was a god, the longest lab coat in the room, if people were measuring. His authority and the respect he commanded from the cloud of residents and fellows around him was clear, my kind of guy, curmudgeonly, competent, pissed off that the rest of the world was not keeping up. He looked at the MRI on the screen, scrutinizing the images with a scowl. "There's nothing there." I was confused. "There's no infarct. The MRI is clean." The grand old man explained to his short-lab-coated protégées what was real and that the anonymous radiologist either did not know his trade or had made a mistake in haste.

When this information reached the other doctors that had become a part of my life, general practitioner and neurological specialists alike, perhaps four doctors in all, they were quick to say, "I'm so glad. I never saw anything either. I never thought there was an infarct." There were lots of questions on my mind: *Why were you treating me for something you did not think I had? Why didn't you look for what was actually wrong if you believed the present diagnosis was baseless?* Their reliance on concept and authority trumped their desire to help or even refrain from injuring a patient with bad treatment.

What You Can Do

Embrace the Unknown, Accept the Contingent

My trade as a lawyer teaches me to be circumspect and sensitive to new facts, especially contrary facts. If a client asked me if the sun will rise tomorrow or if the Miami Marlins will win twenty championship titles before the New York Yankees win their next one, I will tell him all the reasons it should or should not happen. I might go over historical experience. I will never say it will or will not; I know I am not the force in the universe who gets to say whether this happens. If it is not plainly impossible under our current understanding—which itself is contingent and likely wrong, and will be ridiculous to our progeny fifty years hence—the occurrence or nonoccurrence is a matter of likelihood, of confidence always qualified by two very likely truths: 1) We do not know all we think we know, and 2) Often we do not know what we do not know.[4]

---

4.   So you know I try to be fair, here is an example of lawyers, at least formerly, thinking they know everything. At the dawn of my legal career, a massive problem was managing the chaos caused by old film and television agreements that dealt with all the media and modes of distribution known on the Columbia lot circa 1945 or even 1975 but that said nothing about home video, then DVDs, screenings on airplanes, digital distribution, and who knows what else. This was the future, the dawn of the CD-ROM multimedia age! Now I, and I think any good lawyer in the field, would make the territory the "universe" or the "world" if they wanted everything. They would have a license cover "all media now known or hereafter devised" and so on. A generation of entertainment lawyers was fed on the inability of prior generations to contemplate anything other than movies and television.

Raw science research and engineering work, as opposed to the homespun traditions in the clinical practice of medicine, speak in terms of hypotheses and probabilities. All ideas, even from the greatest authority, even Einstein's work, are provisional and need to be proven over the decades with repeated consistent results. (Sometimes Einstein has been shown to be wrong.) We always know that we do not fully know because that is the logical stance and what all of history shows. Human knowledge has not ended. Understanding grows. Anyone who says we know all there is to know about something is a fool. Behind the smallest, most fundamental unit of matter will be smaller things composing that unit that we just cannot see yet. There may be hidden universes in your shoelaces.

Always observe with the understanding that there are contingencies and that unknowns abound. Never let what you see gel into a rigid idea. At that point, you stop seeing.

Stick to What You See

You should never substitute what you see for what someone else sees. Your observation of the world is critical, essential to living in the world. I see this distortion, as discussed, starkly at play in the medical establishment's organizational failures, love of process, and obsequiousness to a hierarchy that they value more than a patient's health or even life. People who know more or have seen more should be given a special audience, but the renunciation of what one sees can never be accepted. This has profound moral and social consequences beyond your own happiness.

There is a wonderful *Star Trek: The Next Generation* episode where Captain Picard is captured by some baddies with a lot of latex appliances on their foreheads. He is tortured and questioned Stasi style, an interrogator wearing him down over days of mind-altering torture, reward, punishment, and interviews. The interrogator merely wants the brave captain to tell him that there are five bright lights shining in his eyes when there are four. The issue in isolation is irrelevant and unimportant. Yet the captain suffers through excruciating torture for refusing to mouth the words "There are five lights." The wise captain knows, as soon as you put faith in someone's word over what is plainly before your eyes, the notion of truth and everything that flows from it is lost.[5]

We cannot reject what we see because someone in authority—a boss, an authoritarian political leader, someone better educated, anyone with a rank one is supposed to follow—says it is otherwise. Education, knowledge, experience, judgment, and perspective are important and should be heard. They should inform your thinking. You will need to rely on experts who can see and understand things you do not, for which you do not even have the basic vocabulary. Do not operate on yourself. Do not ever represent yourself in a legal proceeding. Most folks probably should never even do their own taxes. Know that you do not know. However, substituting your own experience with that of another not for substantive but for procedural reasons denies the validity of your own experience and in doing so gives unlimited power to the person in authority.

This phenomenon is often discussed in the context of the authoritarian impulse in political history. This deference to what the leader says over what plainly happened, what people saw, is the bedrock of Nazism, Stalinism, and many of the hugely bad things in history. They are present in our normal lives and writ large in the context of hospitals and clinics. Sure, there are reasons for clear hierarchy and responsibility in business, including the medical business. The question is whether the hierarchy is tethered to the shared goal (healing a patient or providing better IT support) or primarily exists to perpetuate its own existence.

The psychosocial petri dish of perception and behavior is on display everywhere. It leads to the core questions:

Are we following facts or a characterization of facts?

Are we following what we observe or refusing to accept things we see because someone with greater authority has already told us those things are not there or should not matter?

---

5.   I realize this is a riff on the far more literary example in Orwell's novel *1984* of 2+2=5. There were no spaceship battles in *1984* nor color-coded uniforms featuring go-go boots, so advantage *Star Trek*.

Are we viewing the world through the same misguided lenses?

Is it even possible to see things clearly given our social context?

Learn to Hold Your Hypothesis Loosely

There is no hard-and-fast solution, only a continuing process of observing diligently, being aware of all the things that may be distorting your vision, and learning more concepts and words, while always looking for yourself.

Currently and finally correctly, after many years of medical inquiry, I think, I have learned I have Parkinson's disease. Interestingly, this is an elusive, little-understood disease. It could be a problem of the gut or the brain. There is no objective test—well, not for the living. Once you are dead, they can cut your brain in half and see what was going on. (When they slice my brain open, I hope someone organizes a reveal party.) However, this is the best organizing concept to date. My symptoms fit. There are odd globs of protein associated with the disease that have been shown in biopsies of my leg. It is not a conclusive diagnosis, but it has a huge probabilistic impact. I fit the profile. Every known test and observation are consistent.

That said, I hope I continue to keep my eyes on facts, to observe what is happening with me, always assessing, always examining, prepared to modify my understanding to fit facts and not vice versa. I am proceeding with care on the working hypothesis that I have Parkinson's disease. There is no downside and a great deal of potential benefit, regardless of whether or not I have Parkinson's disease.

I know there are a lot of internal forces driving me toward the concept over fact. Those forces are not what most people would assume. I do not resist the diagnosis. I am not looking for facts to feed a belief that it might not be true. The problem I face is, looking at things with a tight scope, I want to have Parkinson's disease. I want a solid understanding of things. It is comforting and begins a new stage from looking to treating. Believing I have Parkinson's disease is a balm. I am happy to know and feel rather lucky that the expected bad news is just Parkinson's disease. Every medical setting I enter is full of people having much worse days than mine.

I like and respect my doctors, but I also know the last doctor always appears to be the smartest. Both my experience and my learning have shown that both the doctor and the patient have a bias toward a conclusion.

I will do my best to observe what is happening to me, rather than catalog what I see as symptoms of Parkinson's disease. Every hour I find myself falling into the trap. I see my tremor and say, "Ah, that is a symptom of Parkinson's disease and lines up with what I read in a book about Parkinson's disease, confirming everything I know in a tidy circle." I lose my balance a bit, something previously seen as unimportant, but it now becomes a symptom of Parkinson's disease and a subtle entrenchment of operating conclusions.

The diagnostic process for Parkinson's disease has shown me just how difficult it is to see what is happening, because we only look at things we think might be relevant. I have lots of photos of my eyes going wiggy, diaries of the circumstances when I got dizzy. The information I had collected was generally irrelevant. My symptoms are different from and weirder than what I would have imagined. When I write (or could write) the letters got smaller as I went, and the line drifted down and to the right. When I walk, one of my arms does not swing. I have dreams where I have to fight to protect my family, and while I am holding my own, I can never land a clean shot and feel frustrated. They were things I did not know I did, because in my world of concepts and words, they were not things. They were not germane to anything. These irrelevancies not worthy of notice are all symptoms of Parkinson's disease and important to its diagnosis.

The problem is largely one of language. I am not or not yet in the language/thought culture of Parkinson's disease. Neurologists, I am sure, have a word for not swinging one arm, but I do not. Swinging one arm when walking literally was not in my vocabulary and therefore not observed. If I ever noticed it, I would consider it unimportant, information taken in unnecessarily and flushed from memory immediately.

It would be facile just to say, "Keep your eyes and mind open," and move on to the next chapter. The human retina transmits information to the brain at roughly the same rate as an Ethernet cable. We need concepts and language not just to communicate but to make sense of what we see and hear. We cannot pay attention to everything.

Organizing concepts and words are essential. I really need to have a lot of words and concepts to write this or even navigate my way into my office, turn on the lights, sit in a chair, and type. We need words and ideas to guide us to know what sense information should be observed and made the object of contemplation and communication.

This is the conundrum. We move through the world entirely reliant on concepts and language, yet I am arguing that the goal is to see things without concepts and language. I am surely a hypocrite of some sort for communicating this in language. I do not think the situation is a hopeless paradox, however. The task is not to fight against language per se, but interposing language between the world and what you see. The challenge is to turn language off so you can see what your eyes actually see, feel what your skin touches, smell the molecules in your nose, and taste the molecules on your tongue. Then go through your catalog of concepts and words to make sense of it, always holding out the fact that there are not words and ideas to explain most of what happens, always understanding that what you see is contingent and necessarily shaped by everything around you.

However simple this is, it is hard to do, and moving toward it requires practice.

CHAPTER 5

Seeing without Ourselves

We see the world through a haze of stories and biases that we have created and ultimately consider our identity.

A static idea of who you are is, accordingly, a distorting filter that makes clearly seeing things impossible.

To see the world as it is, you must divorce yourself from it.

To see the world as it is, you must accept change, which means you will have to accept new facts and reject things that are no longer true.

To see things as they are, you must continually abandon who you are. Removing self from the equation creates a better self.

Even if one can punch through the veil of concepts to see facts as they are or at least as we sense them to the extent possible, a greater challenge awaits: seeing facts objectively without an idea of self in the way.

To see clearly, we must be willing to see and accept things as they are even if doing so requires us to abandon who we are. This is not easy.

Acceptance of things as they are requires constant and ruthless examination of one's own thoughts. Seeing the world clearly and accepting facts may require that we reject long-held expectations or aspirations. It may even demand that we abandon important notions about our own identity. This is painful, pitting the value of achieving a real life in the world working toward real goals against the value of the many fantasies that bring us comfort and tell the story of who we are, the essence of our identity.

We Are a Distorting Filter

Each one of us is an amalgamation of points of view, biases, explanations, and other stories we tell ourselves, both as individuals and as part of a collective. Anything that could be prefaced by "I believe" would be in this bucket we view as "self." Without the points of view, or biases, and stories about what we have seen and even things we have not seen but wish to believe, many people would fear that they are not in the picture. People legitimately fear that without these fantasies and biases, a human would just be an orb of sensors and memory recording data from the sensors—more or less a computer, and not a smart one. These biases and stories that comprise identity are an internal language that helps people build a model of the world in their minds, providing shortcuts, good or bad, that make navigating the world simpler.

We have strong motives for wanting to believe that we are firmly planted in whatever is happening and, equally important, that we have a substantive identity to assert in whatever is happening. We do not want to die. We want to live. We fear letting go of this. We fear change. We fear becoming nothing, so the mind will concoct rationales, stories, and other devices to distort our view or interpretation of events to fit what we want to believe, to match our biases and bolster the things with which we identify.

Choosing the fantasies that compose individual identity over reality, however, comes at a great cost. Proceeding based on wishes and ignoring disruptive facts makes seeing the world and moving forward toward real-world goals in the real world impossible. Building an identity atop falsehoods threatens consumption with meanness, isolation, even madness. A self either in conflict with known reality or one that distorts reality to keep itself alive results in a destructive instability of mind.

There is a great enemy within.

Attachment to Group Identity

The idea of removing one's "self" from the picture sounds very Zen, something incomprehensible on its face. However, there are practical examples of identity in conflict with reality everywhere, and moving away from fantasy and toward reality is feasible if we are aware of the potential distortions we wish to avoid.

Identity lives in the pieties and biases we have. Personal belief and association is identity. The inability of many people to see or adapt to contrary facts is the source of all the conflicts that make no sense to someone whose identity is not wrapped up in those things. Why do Hutus murder Tutsis? An American observer may be perplexed because they are both "Black." Historically speaking, it seems only natural to an American that a person should be defined primarily by skin pigment. Once you have some distance from it, cultural bias can seem bizarre. Why did a third of Europe destroy itself in fights between Protestant and Catholic ideologies, fights based on differences that seem petty to most schoolchildren when they learn about the seventeenth century today? And why did the English and Irish hate each other? The modern American and someone from a culture more removed, say, an average Korean citizen, are likely to be confounded by the question. Are they not the same thing, the same country even? The accents are different? Really? Is that why they hate each other? Ah, we are back to the Protestant/Catholic thing, aren't we? But is it not the case with religion that the important distinction is which countries are Christian and which are Muslim? What is it with soccer fans fighting each other and tying political and ethnic loyalties to sport? Most of the men actually playing the game are from other places and may be equally perplexed as to how their chasing a ball translates into ethnic, religious, and political hatreds?

Authoritarian figures like Mussolini or, more recently, Donald Trump make loyalty a core pillar of identity. Seen this way, the purported Nazi quote as relayed by Peter Drucker, the postwar business guru, makes sense: "We don't want lower bread prices, we don't want higher bread prices, we don't want unchanged bread prices—we want National Socialist bread prices!" Good, bad, up, down, more, less; these things are irrelevant. The essence of the matter is loyalty. The content of the message is irrelevant. It is the black shirt or the brown shirt that matters. Recently in the US, the same quote was rewritten in the 2020 Republican national platform. The entirety of the platform was a resolution that "the Republican Party has and will continue to enthusiastically support the president's America-first agenda." In other words, whatever Father Leader says now or in the future is what we believe. People who read the "we want whatever we are told to want" platforms of the Nazis, the GOP in 2020,[6] or any authoritarian group, powerful or petty, and see illogical, circular nonsense are missing the essential point of the statement—identity. Whether it's a flag, a jersey, or any other distinguishing characteristic, it sends the message. The content is not important. The identification is the goal and the end.[7]

---

6.   Can you imagine the 1860 Republican platform stating "Slavery? I don't care. Whatever Lincoln wants to do is fine."

7.   This is personal to me. I was an avid Reagan Republican. The ideas were important, rooted in sound theory and values. There was an opportunity to break the old welfare state paradigms that failed to bring everyone up to their full potential. The search for liberal, free-market solutions was where the intelligence and creativity in political ideas rested. Many of the ideas failed, but the outlook and impulse can still do good. Sadly, the GOP is no longer a party of ideas. It is now a party of identity—white; Christian native; male; in hostile opposition to women, minority groups, and immigrants, who they fear will replace them. Loyalty to one man is the uniting belief. The meanness, falsehoods, and hostility to long-treasured ideas and institutions from the leader are not bad, nor are they good, nor are they beliefs, as the leader may change his views instantly. They are tests of loyalty. The more outrageous the conduct of the leader, the more the leader separates the truly loyal from the sunshine patriots. Fortunately, good ideas will endure until sanity returns, or so I want to believe.

A hopefully more muted and, for me, viscerally understood form of identity is sports loyalties. I love my baseball team, the Dodgers. I have passed down this love to my child. We memorize and revere things that happened before we were born. We fetishize any connection to the past. We view Dodger Stadium as hallowed ground. In quiet moments after a game, when there is a serenity, the vibrant green of the field tended by the grounds crew, the scoreboard that displayed a sheet of zeros that night Sandy was perfect, in the same place I saw all my childhood heroes, we weep and embrace. We read and listen to hundreds and hundreds of hours of content, probably more than five hundred hours, per year, texting back and forth and sharing articles, all about guys wearing one jersey, messing with a ball. In the offseason we are like junkies deprived of a fix, and we have much less to say to each other. To what are we really enthralled? What really is the content of this identity that is so central to our lives? Players? It cannot be. They come and go. They retire. They leave and start wearing the uniform of a rival or come from a rival. Owners? There have been good and bad ones, families, corporations, investment groups pursuing different ends. Values and philosophy? The Dodgers have more of an ethos and ethical history than most other teams, but meh. There probably are not too many fans left who feel the brotherhood of 1955 or even remember how Fernando united Angelenos. In the end, what is left is a logo, supporting marketing, and a mythology crafted by brilliant sports writers over the decades. When the logo or location changes, the loyalties change. How many people in Brooklyn are Dodgers fans? I have never met one, but I have met many New Yorkers and descendants of New Yorkers who inherited an ancestral hate for the Dodgers for leaving.

My daughter hates a player from the Mets, an extraordinary, sure-to-be-in-the-Hall-of-Fame pitcher named Jacob deGrom. He is an ace of aces, and I would shriek with joy to see him with "Dodgers" spread across his chest. To my daughter, he is evil incarnate, something inherently wrong, a presence that should not be normalized. When she was about twelve, after I had replaced Barbie and Monster High dolls in her room with the Boys of Summer and bobbleheads of Pee Wee and Jackie, when we started to make our relationship center largely around baseball, the Mets knocked the Dodgers out of the playoffs. DeGrom was masterful, and my daughter learned for the first time that your team does not always win, even when you think they should. It broke her heart, and she may never forgive deGrom. She created an entire villain's backstory for him, which involves him murdering penguins. Wow. That is really a bad guy. She is now a young adult but still carries the animus.[8] Every year I ask her if she would be happy to have deGrom come to the Dodgers. She says, "No! Never!" It could be the best Giant, our perennial foe; the best Yankee, our ancestral foe; but not deGrom, an innocuous Met. Never. There is some humor in the matter now. She gets why it is silly, but she really actually hates this guy for having the audacity to be great while not wearing the logo with which we choose to identify. When I ask, what if he does join the Dodgers? He is about to be a free agent and is a prize. Cognitive dissonance. Something you hate, part of something you love? Imagine Captain Kirk saving a civilization by posing a paradox to a computer, making the computer destroy itself in confusion, with sparks and steam filling the room. (Why are the computers always steam powered?) I love the stories and the traditions, the mythology, the living links to the past, but this is mythology, and the only thing that links us to that mythic past, much of which I personally remember now, is the logo and a very few individuals who may still live but are no longer regularly present.

During games, when I am grasping in anguish at the little hair I have left, praying to every deity I can think of, I always notice how the players generally see each other as human beings. They are old colleagues and friends from other teams, the minor leagues, or youth teams. Even in the most tense, most important World Series games, they are chatting and laughing. They have worn a lot of different jerseys. They know they may be teammates again. They may be going to a wedding of a common friend. Maybe they will be training together in the offseason. They are not the logo. They try their best, and they love the game. The game is the constant for them. Real life. Meanwhile, fans like me, people not playing, just observing with a raw desire, are literally screaming and crying or high-fiving strangers. (At no other time

---

8. I can have no hard feelings toward the Mets logo. When I see it, I see the Dodger blue they imitate, and I remember 1988. Even though I am not religious, I thank all the gods, goddesses, fair folk, and life forces for that year.

am I likely to hug a stranger with a neck tattoo in Gothic letters.) The blind, uncontrollable passion belongs to those of us whose loyalty is to the logo, people with no objective interest in the outcome, people with no control or agency of any kind, mere passive observers. We are so fervent, irrationally, insanely committed, because there is no content to our loyalty. It is a raw identity that we must defend. If the Dodgers lose, we lose. It is powerful and dangerous because its strength is not tethered to any value or idea.[9]

Many European countries have banned the wearing of political uniforms. They know that the power of identification when people are wearing the same shirt is too much for the human psyche to manage. They have seen what it does.

The building blocks of identity are strewn everywhere, with all their dangers and hostility on display. The problem—left or right, this team or that—is always the same. People make these things a staple of their identity, their sense of self. From that point on, they either cannot see contrary facts or must discount or distort them to preserve that sense of self. Only negative things are seen in hated minority groups. One tribe must kill another. Reality be damned, great opponents must be penguin killers.

Attachment to Internal Identity

Those of us who have had the good fortune to have an education or life experience that has resulted in a broader view may have a smugness. We read contrary things and work to sort out incongruities. We know

---

9. The only participant in the game I know of who put logo first was Dodgers manager Tommy Lasorda. He would fight with fans of opposing teams if he thought they desecrated the Dodgers logo. He tackled the Phillie Phanatic mascot for disrespecting the Dodgers. He bled Dodger blue. God was the big Dodger in the sky. Lasorda's casket lay in center field when he died, carried out by the aged members of his great teams of the 1980s. As an adult, I view his loyalty as close to insane. He was an entertaining, wonderful, colorful figure who added a great deal to the game himself and was responsible for bringing great players to the game, but tackling a guy in a mascot suit because he stomped on a hat with your company's logo? Fun, but bonkers.

that flags and arm bands are dangerous and believe we are not prey to such simple misdirection. An appeal to our groupthink passions does not define us or move us. We love our team, but we also know it really does not matter and the team we love is nothing more than a trademark worn by a rotating group of professionals. We can do it with humor, and with a dash of irony too. We can pray at our church and consider the mosque down the street equally valid, because we also recognize it is all fundamentally nonsense or more or less the same wine in different bottles if we are especially fond of what the imams and priests are peddling. We want substance, not slogans. We want facts and reason, not faith. To the extent we associate with one group or another, we hold that identification loosely as a choice among many equally valid options. We do not build our identity on racial, religious, national, or any other group identity, or at least we so tell ourselves.

We should not be too smug. Those of us with a broad, ecumenical point of view are, hopefully, less likely to be genocidal maniacs than others. Group identity is just not strong enough in us to inspire murder. This is something, but it does not mean we see the world for what it is. The stuff above is the crudest, broadest form of identity based on adherence to a group often coupled with hostility to another group, which quite often is exactly the same thing just branded differently. Our sense of self lies in much subtler, internal recesses that require a greater vigilance and ruthlessness to find and remove. Any belief that we have already transcended the brown shirt or flag or religion is itself an impediment to be defined and excised. We must see the buckets in which we place ourselves, the organizations and brands with which we identify, so we can remove ourselves to a clearer vantage point.

Attachment to Our Stories about the World

Our identity also lives within us in the stories we tell ourselves about the world. You could call it viewpoint, outlook, conclusion, predilection, or even wisdom, but the essence is the same. We tell ourselves broad stories about what the world around us is and how it works. Our identity is embedded in our adherence to those stories. We tell ourselves something like people are generally selfish and terrible. Charity is rare, and if you tease it out, you will find the selfishness and terribleness of people even in charitable acts. Or we believe fame, wealth, and other things society values are mirages. Everyone really just wants to be loved. We believe faith is what matters, or faith is an opiate of the masses foisted upon them by the Man. History is a function of economics and class. History is a function of powerful individuals. No, history is the product of competing ideas. No, surely history is an expression of climate, geography, and population change, and so on. All these things are doubtlessly true some of the time. Seeing when one idea or another fits a body of facts is analysis. Believing something as a baseline worldview is, in effect, a religion that serves as a pillar of identity as surely as the outward-looking association with a religious group does.

If I believe people are terrible and generally out to get me, it will color the way I view others. I will be prone to distort what I see to fit that article of faith. I might discount acts of kindness or assume there is some selfish sub-rosa motive. I will cling to facts that support my view and find some way to discount or ignore others. I bring this belief wherever I go, and it necessarily filters facts into good and bad, accepted and rejected. The belief itself may be a distorting lens that moves focus or the interpretation of what we see altogether. The belief is a key part of who we are. It is something we carry and insist upon, separate from any particular facts.

If we believe people are inherently, irretrievably selfish and transaction oriented as a major life understanding, seeing acts of selflessness and caring is problematic. To remain who he is, the cranky man who does not think much of people must reject or diminish those acts. This, like any denial of reality, sets us on a course plotted in a fictional universe of our own making and will not help us do things in the real world or find a stable sense of being.

If we are to see things clearly, we must accept contrary facts, even if they undermine the core beliefs that define us. Looking at the world clearly requires a willingness to destroy oneself in the pursuit of our goals. It takes courage. It takes a high level of mindfulness to sort out the bias from what is actually seen. It is hard. It takes a resolve and ruthlessness.

Attachment to Stories We Tell Others

Who am I? I'm the guy who broke his front teeth in a tragic skateboarding accident in the first grade; who brought fifty-three live chickens to his last day of high school, one for each senior; who played at the Stanford Mausoleum with the Sarcastic Fringeheads on Halloween; who went to school here and there and worked here and there with a shifting body of morality and amusing tales from each stage; who had this friend and that; who did regretful but sometimes hilarious things in nightclubs in Hollywood as a young man; and so on. These events happily recalled years on end, grow in the early years, leaving stagnant middle age and beyond to rehash them. Childhood, adolescence, professional life, married life—all of it is a small body of stuff. There are probably just a few dozen stories I retell regularly and fewer than a hundred major life stories I tell in total.

Our actual stories define who we are. They are even more essential to our definition of self than group identity. Where the group identity drops in a ready-made bucket of attributes that go along with the religious, political, sports, and other brands one chooses to wear in life, the stories are unique to one person. There is not a lot of variation in stories or human experience among most people. The time, technology, economy, civilization, and other tent-pole determinants of history put most people born into them on one of only so many life paths. Still, in the living, each life is unique, even if very, very similar.

The raw experience, however, is not the real locus of our identity, our self. The definition of the self we wish to present to others exists in the stories we tell. The stories are different from raw experience.

Our conscious selves that we wish to present to the world as ourselves are the characters we place in our stories. Some stories are shared with others, but the selection and the entire collection, as well as the point of view and choices in retelling are unique. It is our singular experience distilled down into what matters to us. That is, the things that continue to define us long after the events themselves have passed.

Attachment to the Stories We Tell Ourselves

Our identity is rooted even more delicately and perniciously in the stories we tell ourselves about ourselves. This is paradoxical, but we are largely who we tell ourselves we are. Behind the stories we tell others to place ourselves in the world are stories we tell ourselves. These internal stories may be impacted by the repetition of stories told to others in a feedback loop, but there is necessarily a great deal more behind a story we package and tell others than the story we convey. We need to tell ourselves stories about who we are before we can distill information and construct it into a tale for others. The stories we tell ourselves usually do not contain characters or plot. Rather they are a collection of values and points of view, influenced by, but ultimately independent from, experience and memory. This is bedrock identity, the storyteller trawling through experience, live and in memory, to create and then recount a story about himself.

The storyteller, this idea of self, is itself a concept necessary to function and make sense of the world and, like all concepts, risks distorting the world to support itself. We need an internal storyteller for our internal intellectual life to go on. Our senses take in more than we can remember. We need an arbiter to determine what to tuck away in memory. We do not remember or recall raw sense data. It would be unintelligible. We remember what we think we need to remember in a form salient to the purpose for which we are remembering it. Even if there is no conscious awareness of this happening, it is happening. Choices are being made every moment if not autonomically, then according to some implicit value system. There is a storyteller we create, an identity that chooses what memories to make, how to shape them in memory, how to spin them into a story, and when to deploy that story.

To the extent we have choice in the matter, we tell ourselves who we are and from there cherry pick the memories and bend them into colorful tales both hilarious and terrible. It is this arbiter of memory and spinner of yarns that defines us.

The Stories We Tell Others Place Us in the World

I tell my taking-fifty-three-chickens-to-school story to reinforce to

myself and convey to others that I am a whimsical, irreverent soul looking for comedy, not drama. As I go through life, I collect memories and
construct more stories to support this view. At some point, in some way,
I decided that that was who I was. It is essential to my idea of who I am.

When it comes to running, I believe that I am a terrible runner,
sloth-like in speed, prone to injury, undisciplined when it comes to
doing less, and too aggressive in my efforts to do more. I am old, brit-
tle, struggling to do what is natural and easy for people twenty years
older than I am. Even more specifically, I do a terrible job of managing my bladder on race day, and I am prone to carry too much stuff.
Other runners on race day are generally friendly and supportive where
people in all other contexts outside of running are generally terrible
and proof that the dogs should take over. Most of these things may be
true—they have the ring of lessons learned from discernible facts; then
again, by definition, they would. This is who I believe I am, so these are
the stories I have playing in a useless feedback loop.[10]

This recursive process may be the ultimate seat of identity, but at
root, it is a basket of biases pushing one to sift through experience,
looking for evidence in support of the bias. These values and view-
points that define us to ourselves, our internal editor and author, are
biases designed to distort reality, to push the world into something we
find important or interesting as judged by our internal concept of self.
As such, we are our own worst enemy.

Seeing the world without oneself in the picture is as tall an order
as seeing without any other governing concept. Self may be the ultimate organizing principle we lean on. It takes discipline and dogged
effort to see things clearly. I must continually revisit the search for
sub-rosa biases. Am I focused on observing this pain in my leg because
it is significant in present, actual experience, or am I observing it because I know I am prone to injury? It is hard to see what is happening
without a filter of identity or personality.

---

10. Such beliefs, if true, hold great value. If I know I made a mistake, I can work to
     avoid that mistake in the future. The key here is knowing if the belief is true.
     Constantly revisiting what one sees and thinks is required to ensure that what
     you tell yourself is solely tempered wisdom and not an expression or fear that
     emphasizes and shapes some facts while ignoring or discounting others.

It is especially hard to see things we do not want to see. Looking at the world, including one's own acts within it, shows a great many things that do not line up with one's self-constructed, guiding identity. I say I am an irreverent person when the context calls for projecting who I am, but I am also moody, pensive, brooding, depressed, repressed, angry, and lots and lots of other things that do not fit with the chicken story or anything I would pull out at a cocktail party or interview lunch to show what an interesting, creative guy I am. Even though I recognize that I am not always the fun guy in the story, this is a cloak I have chosen in some way to wear. It is a great story, and the guy in the story is intelligent and irreverent, someone you would want to know. He just does not line up with the facts of much of my life.

The chicken day did happen, and it was my greatest accomplishment (aside from the birth of my children, etc., etc.), shared with a man I still call my friend almost forty years later. There are more facts supporting a darker, negative character. My presence distorts the exercise of seeing and observing, and the story itself becomes a tool and an end. The chicken story has the power to shape how I see the world, defines in part my place in the world and how I move through the world.

While on some level it is impossible to remove yourself completely, it is possible to improve. Instead of a recursive loop of distorting reality, you can run yourself through continual checks on what and how you are seeing, searching for bias. This takes work, real discipline, and focused effort. It is not how we ordinarily live.

It also takes extraordinary courage because much of what we see will not fit within the biases and distortions that we call home, that we call "me." One level is technical. Are our sensors seeing everything and are we processing its relevance objectively? Another level is literally self-destructive. You will always see things that contradict, possibly completely undermine a core myth by which you define yourself. You have to be open to that possibility. You must, therefore, undertake the task of seeing not only without the critical biases comprising self, but with the willingness to alter or discard aspects of your identity.

You have to confront that you are not who you say you are and that the stories from which you emanate are somewhere in between distortions and outright lies. It is not easy.

When Reality Challenges Identity

Strangely, people make the choices that compose their identity and then forget that these were their choices. Our choices can be unmade as well as made and modified as circumstances change. Many people cannot accept the nuance and conflicting signals of reality. It has to be all or nothing. The world must conform completely to an ideal that makes their identity the most certain, unquestionable, best-ever concoction of biases and views.

The Homer versus Reality

This regularly plays out in sports as fans excuse and justify things involving their team and pounce on other teams for the same problems. Many fans are compelled to defend steroids and other drug abuse, cheating, poor stadium safety, and terrible behavior by players when it comes to their team. They bought the hat, and with the hat comes an identity. If the team with which they identify does bad things, that must mean that they are identifying with something that is, in part, bad. That is true, but a step too far for many people. It is too unsettling. It requires too much reflection and willingness to adapt. Fantasies are fed by hometown sports talk radio salving potential dissonance as surely as the stories of a preacher might comfort parishioners in the face of contradictory, ambiguous, or otherwise unsettling facts.

The Republican versus Reality

In my youth, I was drawn to the then new ideas of the Reagan Revolution. Harnessing human nature, which can be acquisitive and selfish, to solve social problems made sense to me. Using government to create economic structures that work and then letting government recede and humans take over seemed more consistent with ideas of liberty than having the government take by fiat property from one group (taxes) and redistribute it to another group (benefits); all the while the dysfunction that created the problems the government seeks to remedy hum along.

My personal assessment with more than thirty years of hindsight is some ideas worked, some did not. A lower-tax, lower-regulation environment may foster growth. However, not all boats rose with the tide. Wealth disparities have increased to levels that make me think about the French Revolution, not the 1950s. There was no trickle down. The Laffer curve was a laugh. Government revenue did not increase either as the pie grew. The Republicans who rode the conservative wave to office on these ideas practiced the opposite once in power, simultaneously multiplying deficit spending while cutting and cutting and cutting the tax obligations of the wealthy class that was receiving the fruits of the growing economy. The stock market has performed miserably under Republican leadership. The median performance of the S&P 500 under Republicans since 1929 is –8.8 percent, with an average of –1.2 percent. For Democrats, the median is 19.7 percent, with an average of 14.2 percent. Republicans increase the deficit. Major tax cuts have not paid for themselves. Cutting taxes cuts revenue. Those are facts. I may have thought there would be a different result, but the numbers are indisputable. However, if I point out these truths to those who identify as Republican, usually I am met with defensiveness, accusations of heresy, even hostility, and this is hardly personal stuff. This is economics data, but once a person identifies with it, as distinguished from agreeing with it, it may be too much, require too much self-examination and criticism to challenge it. Tax cuts pay for themselves. Republicans govern with spending restraint. Increasing the wealth of the wealthy is good for the middle class. The markets love Republican leadership. These things are no longer arguable facts, so they become dogma to the faithful. Stating facts contrary to dogma is heresy, and tempers run too hot for conversation for many otherwise sane people. Again, these are merely policy ideas, not even ethics, religion, or something else where tempers are likely to flare. Even things that are objective and remote are too critical to identity for many people. Sadly, the positive potential of new ideas is suffocated in the cradle. If bad ideas are pursued as dogma, there is no room to let in new, better ideas.

When forced to choose between reality and comforting falsehoods, they choose falsehoods.

The American versus Reality

One of my favorite lawyerish quotes is the old saw by John Adams, "Facts are stubborn things; and whatever may be our wishes, our inclinations, or the dictates of our passion, they cannot alter the state of facts and evidence." He represented the British soldiers tried for committing the heinous attacks of the "Boston Massacre." There really was no "massacre" by any standard definition, and those soldiers were on any read of the facts acting in self-defense, trying to save their own lives. An angry American mob surrounded and attacked the soldiers at the outset. The hostility of the mob created the situation that resulted in the British soldiers killing civilians. John Adams was a reflective, intelligent guy. He was able to say to himself and the world, "I am a patriot to the cause. I may even be president one day. I hate the king's decree. I hate how the British soldiers oppress and humiliate us. One day, if diplomacy fails, I will fight them to the death. Today, in reality, these particular British soldiers, in this instance, are okay guys who were mistreated by our compatriots." Americans attacked the British soldiers. That is a fact. Facts did not matter to those who wanted vengeance against the British. Fealty to their broader ideas and identity called for the sacrifice of truth and justice. Saying, "The British army is terrible to us, but these particular British soldiers did little wrong, and it is possible for our side to do bad things to British soldiers" was too nuanced, a step too far for many people. It undermined their identity. Their identity was as rigid and unchanging as the colors on the flags created to represent their loyalties.

Own False Identity

Little things can be unsettling. In some circumstances, I like to think of myself as a really tough, aggressive guy. Sometimes I like to present myself as a tough bastard ruthless attorney. I even have some stories to support this version of myself, but though factually true, the identity the stories support is false. I hate conflict. I hated being an attorney because sometimes it required me to do tough-guy, combative things, and I found it so distasteful I would end up in the hospital from stress-related ailments—heart, head, gut, you name it. I picked the wrong profession. I also know that I pull out this totally off-base identity when I feel insecure. I retreat into it, despite its falsehoods, and the cost of saying I am a tough person who does not care if he is liked is that when I deploy these stories, I do not end up being liked. I am insecure in some social situations, but not adversarial, and I generally like people. I have never embraced an identity encompassing these truths.

To some extent, I have been a tiny bit of a tough guy, but in a pitiable sort of way. I am a little psycho when it comes to physical challenges. I will risk significant pain and personal injury to make a point. For whatever reason, I have had a tolerance, physical and psychological, for physical pain. I do not feel or properly read the pain signals that tell a well-functioning person to stop. In high school, going psycho in sports was a part of this identity. My failing in combat sports was being both bad and unwilling to accept loss, ever.

I tried judo in college for a few years. It was a club sport, not NCAA, so I think they had to let me in. In true Stanford fashion, the coach was the US Olympic coach. There were maybe a dozen regulars, including aspiring Olympians. Other kids were lifelong judoka who had competed since childhood. I believe there were students in the club who had spent time at intense judo schools in Japan. There was an extraordinary guy who pioneered judo as a sport for the blind. And there was I—a mediocre high-school wrestler and only that good in the smallest schools' division. I had never done judo. My only legitimate place on the mat was as a beginning student hoping to learn from the better players, privileged to watch and participate with a coach and teammates way, way, way better than I had earned. I, however, wanted to be competitive. Ultimately, this meant I was a practice dummy. I was always hurt, yet unwilling to take a break. Where I would feebly roll a guy at two miles per hour over my hip, my superior practice mate would slam me to the mat so quickly that I did not know I was no longer on my feet until my back and head hit the mat with a hard slap, which is not what is supposed to happen. Where I would be a clumsy ballroom dancer, slowly and ineffectively pushing my opponent into my leg, my opponent would trip me on the fly, instantly catapulting my feet above my head and leaving my shoulder and head to break my fall—again, this is not the way a fall is supposed to happen.

There comes a point where being incompetent at a sport crosses the line from foolish to dangerous. If you have been to a professional baseball game and watched the bullpen, really seen major-league pitching close up, the speed and violent pop of the ball in the catcher's glove is jarring. The ball is alive, scary, with a weapon-like quality to it. It is a vastly different thing from what you and your mates ever did playing as kids. It is a different animal. Such was the difference between my efforts and the results of my peers. I was throwing long, slow, arcing, inaccurate lobs at forty miles per hour, an eephus to baseball nerds. They were grooving ninety-five-mile-per-hour lasers at my head, snapping me to the mat. I did not belong in the same room with these guys as a competitor or even a well-paired practice mate.

The truth is, I really did not want to be in the room. It was my idea of self as a tough guy, a fighter (Ha!) that brought me there. It was never fun due to my unrealistic approach. I never had any aptitude, but I needed to be someone doing something like that to preserve my false face. Once there, a sane person would have taken it easy, and there would be no shame. After all, I was a novice recreational player. The other guys were somewhere between really good high-school competitors and world class. They were all fellow students, all really nice people. Nobody would come close to saying or even thinking, *That Craig is such a pussy. No wonder girls don't like him.* My trying to hang, even in practice, was as absurd as my having a student research assistant or summer associate and expecting them to do the work I can do as a lawyer with thirty years' painful, hyperaccelerated experience. If anything, I would think it was a bizarre character failing and lack of judgment if the student, probably someone thirty years younger than I, insisted on doing work at my level even though they would necessarily fail. This was the same situation, only the cost to me was physical. I was always hurt. I hated it. I should not have been there and did not want to be there, but having been shut out of the other activities that said "tough guy" to me, I could not quit without altering my identity, a very false and wrongheaded identity.

I can laugh at it now, a little. At the time, I was mired in inner turmoil, and this blindness to fact or, in my case, acknowledgment but refusal to accept fact, actually made me much worse at being the "tough guy" I wanted to be. This is another personal example of how refusal to see and accept facts necessarily leads to failure. If I had been focused on becoming a better judoka over the long haul, I would have taken it easy and focused on learning. I would not have been hurt all the time and may have enjoyed myself. I was literally one of maybe fifteen people kneeling at the feet of the US Olympic coach. I practiced with excellent players who were not my competitors and would be happy to instruct me. I chose to stew in anger rather than take advantage of this extraordinary opportunity for a novice to learn.

This character flaw, this clinging to an inapt story of self, had real physical consequences. The most important and the first thing you learn in judo is how to make a safe, good fall. That is the key to everything. Without a safe, good fall, judo is not a sport but a style of fighting that kills or breaks. It is up to the player to decide that his opponent has an effective choke or arm bar, positions that would let him render his opponent unconscious or break the arm, admit defeat, tap out, and end the match. It is up to the player to decide that his opponent is tripping or throwing him successfully, effectively concede on that move, and focus on making a safe fall. I never learned to make a good fall or tap out. My false identity made doing so a form of quitting, and quitting is unthinkable for a tough guy. (Again, to myself, ha!) The thought of tapping out or making a good fall never occurred to me in the moment. I would be stuck in rage and struggle. When I had a conscious thought, it would be something like *I would rather die than lose to this motherfucker.* I would mean it. So I would land on my shoulder rotator cuff instead of my back. I would leap, landing with my full weight on the top of my foot, the toes knuckled under. I would be choked, then wake from unconsciousness with the coach reviving me and the whole club staring at me. It was not smart. It was not learning. It was not having fun.

I was in a fantasy world trying to demonstrate something to myself by trying to do things I did not know how to do and could not possibly do. I was not really trying to learn. I was living in fantasy and trying to achieve a goal generated by fantasy. By living in fantasy and working toward achieving things in fantasy, I missed the opportunities I had in reality. I could have learned so much in that club. Maybe I would have developed a lifelong hobby. I certainly would have been more open to making friends.

I have always been an observant, inquisitive, and reflective person, maybe even more as a youth than now. I cannot claim I was blinded by faith or the circumstances in which I was born. I knew exactly what was happening and what I was doing. I knew I wanted to hone a physically tough image to myself and, if it would ever be possible, the world, because of my own insecurities. I was so deeply shy and unsure. I hated myself so much. I was so depressed and untreated I needed something more than being a good student to counterbalance my vast insecurities and self-loathing. I knew it was destructive. I dreaded going. I hurt. I knew I was doing it solely to maintain an identity that no longer fit, if it ever did. Yet I could not change. In my late teens and early twenties, I could not abandon my fragile sense of self. I was too afraid.

I saw all this clearly yet steered directly into the oncoming, inevitable crash. I was not the person I wanted to be, and I never would be. The facts made that clear. I would have to modify my sense of self or sink ever deeper into a world of delusion and denial. This was not a path to success or happiness. Even if I were able to see clearly in lucid moments, I did not accept facts and proceed based on facts, because doing so threatened my concept of self too much. I was too afraid. I did not know who I would be. I was too afraid to embrace a self that shifts as the world shifts, that is uncertain, entirely dependent. I could not accept that if self existed in any sense, it had to be found within the process of living in a changing world.

The Liberation of Self-Destruction

I may keep returning to this story of the fake tough guy because it relates to an identity mostly abandoned long ago. It is safe to tell the tale. Perhaps the tale itself is an important part of my present identity, the identity of one who examines life and tries to do better. I am not consciously aware of any evasion, but perhaps I'm just playing the game of making positive examination and reflection, destruction of self, a new identity, a new self, and building another fictional story, another rickety bridge over a frightening reality. I am sensitive to the possibility, but I do not think this level of semantic parsing matters.

It is the exercise and its continuation that matter. You will be able to avoid mistakes knowing that you are a person that makes those mistakes. When the mistakes are avoided, you can accept yourself as a person who does not make those mistakes. You will be able to accept the world as something independent from and generally disinterested in your private concept of self and how you choose to operate within and present to the world. Even if the new understandings are incorporated into a sense of self. It is in an iterative process. That identity is held loosely, conditionally, and with the understanding that the aim of the identity is to destroy itself and replace it with a better, more truthful one. Ultimately, hopefully, the concept of self becomes unnecessary. That is the aspiration anyway.

This is a difficult process. Seeing clearly is a radical, self-destructive exercise. Constant attention is necessary, as is a willingness to destroy yourself in search of truth, to sacrifice your identity to see what is actually happening. You have to be ruthless in upending what you think you know and therefore who you think you are. You have to burn the things you cling to, your key stories and the concepts you deploy to organize and understand the world. You must recognize the falsehood, sometimes conscious lies, that define you. This is hard. It is painful. It is unsettling. It is also liberating. It is the only way to escape fantasy and to live and grow in reality.

In return for a willingness to constantly comb through and eliminate elements of your identity, you receive reality and a sense of self that, instead of being cast in concrete as a story that wears down over the years, is recreated daily as part of an ever-renewing process. As soon as you embrace change as a central element of identity, acceptance of reality loses its undermining potential. An identity rooted in reality, always growing and always changing, is more authentic. It lets you see the world and live in it as the world is and as you, in fact, operate within it.

Paradoxically, an examined life premised on the best possible understanding of the situation, devoid of the biases and stories that define us, promises a more adaptable, harmonious, and secure sense of self. It may just be a more impersonal self.

PART III

Increased Suffering: The Price for Avoiding Reality

CHAPTER 6

The Nature of Fear

Fear arises from a failure to see and accept things as they are. It arises because:

> we want to know what we cannot know; or
> we need to make decisions whose outcome is unclear; or
> the world as it is now is not the way we want it to be.

Fear may be part of an entirely internal game detached from reality and any practical objective or real-life connection.

It is a negative emotion, sometimes destructive and always a diversion from the work one should be doing to achieve a goal or happiness in the real world.

A Scary Fantasy with Many Faces

Fear manifests itself in many different ways. If we want to know a future we cannot know, we might say we are anxious. If we fear talking to other people because they might reject us, we might say we are shy. If we are afraid of change or things that seem alien and threatening, we might experience anger. Anxiety. Anger. Shyness. It is all fear by different names.

Fear can be rational and useful. If a bear (or snake) were attacking us, a slug of adrenaline and an immediate impetus to run might be useful, but a situation in which fear is a useful response almost never arises.

We create most fear, anger, and anxiety. These feelings are born of excessive concern with how the future could unfold. They arise from things we do not know or cannot know. They focus on things beyond our control, even things that may exist only in fantasy. They are easy emotions to conjure, and nurturing them is comforting, strangely so given their disruptive and destructive nature.

It is easy to be anxious or fearful even when the actual situation at the time is objectively not at all bad, even good by any objective metrics. Everyone can create a fantasy world they want to live in and be angry that it is not real. Everyone can fear the future if they so choose. Everyone can regret the past. There are endless things in the world to fear, from airplanes falling out of the sky to shark attacks all the way down to an unkind remark. There is a lot about which to worry, innumerable things to fear, including, as Franklin Delano Roosevelt noted, fear itself.

The future is unknowable. We can prefer an imagined world where we are the authors of the fantasy and can create the world we wish, but such an internal fantasy world is not reality. It is a reflecting pool of our familiar prejudices. This narcissistic gaze may actually keep us from seeing a sea of distressing reality beneath the surface, real problems we should address.

There is no end to this path. Fear is a negative spiral down the emotional drain.

These Emotions Are Painful and Destructive

Living with anger, anxiety, and any other emanation of fear is unpleasant for everyone, crippling to some, and for most unnecessary at best. These emotions limit the lives of many people, however they are manifested—fear of leaving the house, shyness, physical insecurity, phobias, and the list could go on. For people who have panic attacks or feel these emotions acutely, even anticipatory anxiety, fear that something will happen to induce panic, can itself be a major limiting factor in life. There can be an intense physicality to these emotions. The body might resort to hyperventilating or a loss of consciousness to manage the intensity of anxiety. Slugs of adrenaline amp the body in the face of fear. Many people earnestly believe they are dying when having a panic attack.

Being fearful, angry, or anxious is not pleasant. These states have the potential to destroy a life through any number of means. They are all variants of pain. They entice people to disengage from reality and what they should be doing to move forward with their lives. Instead of taking positive action in the real world, people are driven by an off-target factual premise and the intense emotion of these states.

Fear-related emotions are concerned exclusively with hypotheticals and keep the mind locked in a world of negative possibilities outside wise consideration of choices to be made and learning from those decisions. Certainly, thinking about possible outcomes in the future is important to making a good decision, as is looking backward to derive lessons from past experience. However, where thoughtful consideration and the objective autopsy of an outcome, good or bad, typically come to an end, fear in its various forms continues into pointlessness and destruction. Fear rehashes the decision even in the absence of new thoughts and information. Fear dwells on mistakes, not to learn, but to generate anger toward oneself, the world, other people, and anything else that that might prevent the desired fantasy world from coming into being.

Because fear's various forms are creatures of an imaged world, sometimes entirely disassociated from reality, indulging them diverts effort from goals and important, real things. Decisions to satisfy fears that are rational solely in delusion are unlikely to be useful or wise. Making decisions to allay fears is choosing to box an imagined opponent instead of the one actually in the ring with you.

Fear, anger, anxiety, and all their cousins can also be destructive. They are negative in orientation and pessimistic in outlook. Seeing enemies where there are none is not a way to make friends or be likable. Being afraid of positive situations keeps one from engaging in positive situations. Dwelling on failure is likely to preclude effort. Fear bypasses examination of good outcomes, as the emotion by its nature lives in the negative. Nobody gets anxious over the possibility of a good outcome. Fear ignores the things that likely lead to success as a result. At best, fear in all its forms pulls us from our actual world into the fantasy in which the emotions swim. They are a source of pain always and total destruction sometimes.

There is good news. Psychiatric disorders aside, fear in all its forms is something we create and therefore can uncreate. So why do we so often elect to indulge in, even nurture, these negative, painful, destructive emotions? Avoiding pain and destruction is neither as obvious nor as simple as it sounds, particularly with respect to anger. People love their fears, anxieties, and anger. They root their identity in them. We identify not as much by our affinities, but by the things we hate, fear, and worry about.

This is insane. It is like jabbing a fork in your eye, understanding that it hurts, understanding the blindness it causes is limiting, but continuing to jab the fork in your eye because you find it is soothing in its familiarity, and however much it hurts, you view yourself as the guy who jabs his own eye with a fork.

Why?

Righteous Anger Is Good or So We Are Taught

Anger is the most common publicly expressed form of fear. Many people love being angry despite its unpleasantness. Anger, even if it is self-destructive, is comfortable. Beyond this we are taught anger is good, and maybe necessary.

Much of the social messaging we receive embraces anger. It is a self-righteous, justified anger that motivates the good fight. Dr. King may have tried to guide us otherwise, but when I think of Rosa Parks and Jackie Robinson disrespected, unjustly attacked, injured, I am angry, and I think of them feeling angry. I imagine, as Hollywood has scripted it many times, that it is their righteous anger that changed the world for the better. It is the hero's hatred of the enemy that fuels his drive to victory. Indignation is our celebrated motivation. We love a fight for what is right. Jackie and Ms. Parks were deservedly indignant. Jackie played with something to prove, absorbing spit and invective from the crowd and taking spikes into his ankles without complaint, quietly waiting for the opportunity to flatten a racist bastard with his halfback skills. Payback. He had to be angry. There is nothing Zen about decking an opponent, nothing serene about revenge. It was a terrible, unjust world, and a giant load of the burden of changing it rested on one man's shoulders. Jackie said he did not need to be liked, but he demanded to be respected. Those are the words of a superhero in Dodger blue, not a passive monk. It is the hero's hatred of the enemy that fuels his drive to victory.[11]

We are rarely told that anger is negative. We are merely taught that anger can be directed or misdirected to good or bad purposes, even though anger is always an unpleasant emotion and distorts what one sees and does.

Anger moves people to good or evil. On the one hand Jackie and Batman, on the other hand every authoritarian leader and comic-book villain. The despot always sits on a foundation of hatred and resentment, even if he has to create fictional enemies to distract people from the fact that their lives are not improving under his rule. Anger at immigrants, the welfare state, wars, peace, trade, lack of trade, and many other potent and important things can motivate anger to the point of murder.

---

11. I cannot claim to be a contemporaneous fan of Jackie. He died when I was three years old, far too young, when he was my age, as I write. I am a fan because he is a hero fueled by righteous anger, anger born of an evil that was not as overt or hopefully strong in my generation. I do try to practice what I write and truly believe, but I love Jackie because the world was grossly unjust, and he fought. I often watch videos of Jackie playing, stealing home in the World Series (Yankee fans, he was indeed safe) and generally being a badass. I have schoolboy fantasies about the Boys of Summer, pretending that they somehow made the world better with a child's game, all unrealistically romantic, I know. I almost never fantasize about or watch videos of Jackie in his suit-and-tie role as a civil rights leader. The injustice, the righteous anger, and the resolution in violence is the appeal. I am not immune.

When large populations identify with what they hate, anger can escalate and remain escalated even in the unspeakable aftermath. Many people blame Jews for their misfortune, even in countries like Greece that have already murdered virtually all their Jews. (Do they need to unearth the corpses and shoot them again just to make sure their solution is final?) I believe Stalin deflected public anger at him, a murderer of millions, by directing anger against an imagined socio-economic class, kulaks, peasants who appeared poor like everyone else but were, in fact, crypto bourgeoisie, invisibly hoarding goods, taking more than their share and therefore responsible for the daily misery of everyone else. Remarkable. Once you have killed every scapegoat, just make up another one.

People Just Love Being Angry

People simply want to be angry. People who have everything, really nothing about which to be angry in their own lives, and do not fall prey to terrible mass delusions find things about which to be angry anyway. No matter how petty or imagined, the anger will rise. In fact, we often cling to anger so long, long after the events that triggered our anger have passed that it becomes an established, permanent hatred that stands alone regardless of facts, no longer something that even has a toe in reality. Hatred becomes a stable crux of our identity.

In my less active days in Memphis, I would go to McDonald's or Starbucks in the early afternoon. Each shop contained the same people in the same general mix—retired white men with nothing to do except sit and drink coffee. (I cannot point too many fingers. I was there too.) The only difference between the two establishments was social class—one group blowing on four-hundred-degree brown water in a large Styrofoam cup, the other sipping a more drinkable brew from a paper cup that is not large, but venti. The conversation was always the same—grousing about how everything was terrible and how much they hated it. It often took the form of senseless invective against people based on ethnicity, religion, belief, and national origin, all the prejudices the Constitution treats as distinctly un-American. Despite the

Constitution, history, and decency, these folks were certain that they were the only good Americans in a world that demanded their righteous anger. It was frequently and loudly stated that Black people are the real racists, and if only Black people had their superb values and were more like them (i.e., more like white people), they would see that there is no racism, just bad, lazy people who happen to be Black. Put differently, these men argued that if only Black people understood that the problem is not white racism against Black people, they would see the problem is that everyone with dark skin was violent and lazy. Oy.

The dynamic was bigger than Southern racism. Anything could be a source of hatred and invective. If I were to lob in a comment like "I don't know why they put out Splenda next to the sugar. Sugar isn't good enough for these people?" or "Why the hell would they change the old cup lids?" or "These paper straws are terrible!" or "Look at that kid's haircut!" then, played right, emotions over those things could run hot.

Black people, Jews, Mexicans, Chinese people, big box retailers, big tech companies, every arm of the government, modifications to Dr. Seuss books, the holiday designs on the Starbucks cups—there are lots of things to hate, and even more petty things to make up to hate. Wealthy, white, male Christians in America, probably the most privileged group in human history, feel aggrieved and put upon, a hated minority in a hostile land. On top of that, the people here sit in a wealthy suburb of a major city. Given the manifestly ahistorical and factual absurdity of their grievance, you have to conclude that people just like being angry at the world. They define their cultural and political identity with hatreds. People with everything are angry that they do not have more. People are angry if someone else has something even if it is much less than they have and does not come at any cost to them. People love their anger and will let go of it more slowly than their affection.

You would think hatred must feel great to have such an allure running against all facts and sanity. Not so. If we can take an objective look, it is clear that however comfortable anger may be, however we may have deployed it in our lives, it is not pleasant. It is not joy. It is not contentment. It is negative and painful not just to others, but to the owner.

Why? Why choose to view a good situation as bad? Why make a tough situation worse? Why not make the journey as pleasant as possible? Why not be happy?

Anger makes us feel right, superior. It makes us feel like we are keepers of some truth. Our masochism is a puzzle and very personal to me.

Anxiety, Stress, and Self-Hatred as a Way of Life and Death

The desire to sustain anger at others is not something I share. If I become angry, I really dislike it and want out. I dislike what it does to me and the people around me. I work to overcome it. For me, anxiety is the problem. Anxiety over the future has made much of my life unhappy. Perhaps the flavor of fear one embraces against all sense is a reflection of personality. My personality directs more toward anxiety and stress.

One can have extreme anxiety over losing identity. If identity is rooted in some fact or performance that is difficult or unpredictable, the fear of change or failure that undermines personality can be intense. I spent my youth with my bowels tied in painful knots, up all night with stress because I might not get an A and, beyond that, lose my identity as one of the smart ones. In fifth grade, I ended up at the UCLA medical center to undergo unpleasant, semioutlandish medical testing. One test required me to eat a radioactive turkey sandwich. I had an instrument and wire shoved up my nose and down my throat, where it stayed for a day. I had dye injected into my kidneys. I had a totally unnecessary appendectomy because I did not have the courage or words to articulate at the time that my bowels were a symptom. The disease was anxiety, stress.

The anxiety got me to Stanford for college and some graduate school (a BA and MA in four years with all the honors and distinctions) and then Harvard for law school (graduating magna cum laude, not super easy), but not without exacting a heavy price—endless stress and unhappiness.

At age twenty-nine as a practicing lawyer, I was blacking out. I was under immense stress, drafting joint venture and licensing agreements that would have a major US ISP and media company bring internet and possibly satellite and telephone services to much of Latin America. I would be working away, nauseous and anxious, and find myself on the ground. Again, I went through the medical wringer, but I knew it was stress. Unable to endure the pressure, I fell unconscious, my body taking over and doing what had to be done because I did not have enough courage to quit or slow down. Same story. My anxiety drove me to collect professional status and titles so that by age forty I felt tapped out, there were no more gold stars to collect. I had everything but felt miserable. My anxiety escalated to the point of no return. Since that time, I have had to make drastic changes in my life. I have been to many good places professionally, always looking for the next, greener hill. I have good places to go, but I do not because no matter what I do, my stress follows me. No, I end up on the floor.

Looking backward, of course, all I see is a misspent youth and needless pain. What narcissistic, silly fears I had that led to hospitals and dry heaving over a toilet seat before school exams. I was so afraid, and there could be no end to the fear, as my ego was tied to being considered among the smart ones in an ever-more-selective group. I could never be done. The stress, over nothing outside my head, really, could only grow. This was my life.

Worry aka the Fool's Gold of Rational Effort

Worry is the devil in the dark.[12] It looks like care and effort, but it is anxiety in a mask.

Worry is in my veins. My grandmother used to pace at night, rattling off her fears out loud in a trancelike state. My mother is likewise an insomniac via worry. There is no unusual fear in our family. We are a fortunate family, upper-middle class, but there are always fears if you want them—unemployment, illness and death, the normal heartaches of love, marriage, and family life, all multiplying as the family grows.

---

12. My fellow Trekkers can hear Spock screaming, "Paaaain," as he melds with the Horta.

Even as a child in suburban privilege, I worried. *What if I get a B? Can I go to the dance considering I'm in the "funny, fat kid" role? Will I make the team, or am I forever cast as the "funny, fat kid"?* The greater my fear about something, the greater my anxiety. Normal social events were a source of anxiety, and I would try to play out every possible scenario in my mind, thinking and rethinking what to wear, how I would say hello to whatever girl I was enthralled with. There were a thousand decisions to make to get to that spot in the gym when I would say hello to the girl . . . *Or should it be "Hey" or "Sup," or maybe I should be really cool and walk by the first time and come back later with a warmer greeting? "Well, hi, howdy do"? No that is not right either.*

My First Marathon: Gargantuan Fear, Endless Variables, Endless Worry

My first marathon was a source of immense worry. I was afraid. The distance remained a mystery. I had invested a great deal of my life, even my identity, in running the 26.2 on that one day. The cost of failure was high, or so it seemed. The more scenarios I imagined, the more possible points of failure I saw.

I could have asthma problems, a real possibility. I could develop a blister and want fresh socks. I could lose a contact lens. Those could really happen too. I could run into nutrition problems. My phone could go dead, and I would not be able to call for a ride at the end of the course, and I would also miss out on taking photos. My watch could die.

I could need water, electrolyte fluid, carbohydrates in various forms. There were dozens of products to audition and endless work to be done to craft the best suite of things to take with me. There are so many choices—gels, tablets, bottles, waffles, bars, cookies—and in so many brands, flavors, and recipes. Also I could get just straight-up hungry.

Which shoe to wear for my big day was a universe of decisions, made increasingly complex by injuries and other difficulties that would pop up unexpectedly in my training. What clothes to wear was a huge matter—compression wear on my calves, thighs, even arms, a hat, sunscreen. I would need warm clothes for the dark hours before the start, but what layers—zip up or pullover?

My stress was too great to contemplate making it the 1.5 miles max to the next aid station. I would take a hydration pack, the largest the company makes, but with what water-to-sports-drink proportions, what extra bottles to carry, and on and on. How to pace myself, how to park, how to change out of cold-weather clothes, how much to run and walk, how to account for the elevation profile of the course, and how to manage my bladder were a constantly shifting body of questions. These unknowns drove me to research and buy a lot of stuff in my quest for answers.

The more I learned, the harder things became. The more I knew, the more there was to worry about. Every book and article I read, however framed, really seemed to be about possible problems, and every problem seemed possible. Nothing was ever decided. Everything was tentative and provisional. This was all new turf. I had no basis in experience on which to rest. All I had was gargantuan fear and a desire to allay my fear by addressing possible problems.

There is a wonderful children's book titled *If You Give a Mouse a Cookie* by Laura Numeroff. It tracks all the consequences that follow from giving a mouse a cookie, consequences of consequences of consequences ad absurdum. If you give a mouse a cookie, he will want milk. If you give a mouse milk, he will want a straw. By the end, the mouse needs tape to hang a picture on the refrigerator, and the original desire for a cookie is long forgotten. That is how my thinking ran.

The upshot is I carried a great deal of food, water, and gear on race day. I had a 1.75-liter bladder of water, 32 ounces of sports drink in bottles in addition, a portable nebulizer with enough medicine to last months and spare batteries to power it, a phone charger, pills and gels and gummies jammed into every pouch, power bars for after the race, spare contacts with contact solution, spare eyeglasses, sunscreen, socks. I had gym bags full of food and other stuff, blankets and pillows to set up the car as my little home before the race. I could have camped out for a few days comfortably in the parking lot. Truly. I carried extra water and sports drink in my hands to the corral (so I would not have to dip into the 102 ounces of water in my pack), wearing enough layers of clothes to keep me comfortable through every subtle change in temperature as the cool night dissolved into a hot morning.

If I worried about something, there was likely a thing I carried the whole run to make me feel that I had it covered. My backpack and the throwaway bottles in my hand weighed over twelve pounds! No joke.

The sense of security from carrying all this stuff was false. Not only was the weight an anchor I had to drag 26.2 miles but the things I carried were not helpful. When things went wrong that day, I had no remedy in my bag of tricks. In my worried state, I could only address the hypotheticals that I could (a) think of and (b) address by researching and finding a solution I could carry. The universe of things that could go wrong was much, much larger and far more unpredictable. You attempt the marathon precisely because it is an odyssey into extremes that will test you in ways you have yet to experience. The things I carried had little likelihood of being useful, and even so, little likelihood of being significantly helpful.

The absurdity of this confounds me even now: I am deeply afraid that I will not be able to run the 26.2 miles. My solution: I will carry an unnecessary twelve pounds. It was fear that drove me to carry 2.5 liters of liquid despite the fact that I would never be more than twenty minutes from water. All the little bits and pieces focused on a thousand discomforts went into a ridiculously heavy pack for 26.2 miles, which itself jeopardized my success.

Why Worry?

The mental and emotional circles of worry help us cope with the discomfort of not knowing what will happen. It is an entirely internal mental game seeking solely to satisfy internal emotions largely detached from reality. It has little to do with rational planning and preparation.

What I was doing was not about the actual failure points of the race, and actually increased my risk of not finishing. Why was I compelled to pursue this energetic, time-consuming foolishness? In truth, I could not deal with the discomfort of not knowing what I could not know. Would I finish? Worry is a manifestation of fear over variables beyond our control. My efforts to address it were detached from the source of the worry—successfully finishing my first marathon.

Many variables are, in fact, unknown, unknowable, or beyond our control. Many of those variables could keep us from achieving our goal. Quite often, things do not go as planned, however good our plan is and however rock-solid our discipline may be. This causes fear. We fixate on one or a few such variables, not as an honest appraisal of the situation, but as a means of creating the illusion that *if only* this or that happens the way we wish or *if only* we get a break on this one variable, everything will be okay.

I was terribly afraid of the race. I did not know how it would go, and I so badly wanted it to go well. There were not many productive things I could do outside of my scheduled training and injury recovery plans. If this took two hours per day, I had another fifteen waking hours to be afraid of the impending trial and nothing useful to do about it. Often, I would have sleepless, worry-filled hours in bed on top of that. In reality, there was not much I could do to perform well. All factors outside the reach of training and diet were unknowable, a void I filled with endless fears and hypotheticals.

Dealing with every imagined contingency displaced some of the fear in the long hours of the day. It gave me something to do, to buy, to read about, to try. I could tell myself I was moving toward the finish line. I could pretend that all would be well if those things were well. Based on that logic, if only I had expanded my kit to twenty pounds I would have so many potential problems covered I could have qualified for Boston!

In fixating on just a few things within your control, you play to your fears, not reality, and therefore, you are not working toward your goal.

Worry Is Unproductive

Worry is a fixation on a specific thing or things. There are a great many things that require effort and attention, not just those within the scope of our worried fixation. Reason, not worry, should direct those efforts. Worry draws attention away from the things we can control and the things we should be doing.

A thousand hours trying to imagine all the possible ways you could fail is unlikely as a practical matter to help. The world is infinitely complex and unpredictable. In truth, there are many things that can go right or wrong, many things beyond the scope of our worry. The things that go wrong are often surprising things we did not worry about or even consider. Almost by definition, if you prepare well, the things that end up being problematic will be total surprises. Your prior weeks of worry will likely be an entirely internal and irrelevant sideshow.

Rational preparation will identify the things that matter, like strength, endurance, and pace. Hours spent designing fail-safe scenarios are probably an exercise in chasing your tail.

The things that have gone wrong for me have always been unforeseen. One year, I had metatarsal pain, a significant soreness on the ball of my foot that had me limping. I had a great podiatrist, a regular Boston Marathon runner who rigged a shoe for me. This let me run but had its own problems on race day. After some miles, all the padding and foam in my shoe compressed, and I was slipping out. I did not foresee that, nor did my doctor. Variable on variable. Those squeamish should skip the next paragraph.

One year I had a massive hemorrhoid two weeks before a race. This was not a mere nuisance. Walking hurt. I had this thing the size of a baby's ear sticking out of me. There was no fix except surgery, which was no help for the race. At no point while auditioning different socks and gels did I think I should spend some time hedging against the possibility of a giant hemorrhoid. Sometimes I have double vision during a race, which makes bumps in the street and curbs perilous. As much as I prepared, as much as I studied the map and had even written out a game plan for each segment, I never paid any attention to bumps in the asphalt and where I might be pushed up and down a curb. More than once, I have come close to falls that would end a race and beyond. (You think I would have learned to walk through the course prior to a race by now.) The things about which I have obsessed, for which I carried gear and read posts and books voraciously, have always been nonfactors.

I was always playing to my fears, and my fears as far as worry goes could not encompass anything but the foreseeable. Problems tend to arise from the unforeseen. Worry was never helpful.

Even if you are worried about something valid and at least partly within your control, the worry is never productive. It adds nothing positive to the enterprise, assuming there is already a desire to do well and to do the things we can do to achieve our goal. Expending mental energy on what we cannot know or is beyond our control is pointless. What is beyond our control is beyond our control.

In my last marathon, I ran with a race belt with gels, keys, credit and insurance cards, a phone, and an inhaler. That's it. I was able to make it to the aid stations. At least I can learn.

Serenity of Race Morning: The End of Worry

In the case of preparing for a race, worry necessarily ends. The thing that generated the worry happens, or at some point close to the event, you realize there is truly nothing that can be done. This end of worry is serenity, equanimity, profound contentment. Streaming fears masquerading as thought gives way to transcendent contentment.

That feeling, the lifting of worry, is one of my favorite things about race day. I have a morning of freedom on the heels of hundreds of days of anxiety and worry, especially if the race is any sort of first for me. It feels like there is so much that could go wrong. As the days to race day shorten and then draw down to hours, everything matters, each bagel eaten, each Gatorade imbibed. There are a hundred little decisions to make, and I have no idea whether they are the right ones. I have a sea of written information, but the lack of independent judgment makes each new article and chat board post an additional problem to sort out. Nothing is known and everything matters. The clock ticks loudly.

Fortunately, the fear usually lifts as I drive in hours before dawn and walk around the starting area. The day has arrived, and there is truly not a thing I can do to change anything as I sit waiting for the hours to go by. I have a feeling of serenity. For the LA Marathon, being in Dodger Stadium predawn, all but alone in the stands, is a dreamlike, quiet experience. At a beach race, the incomprehensibly ancient ocean keeps watch with me. The rhythm of the waves always has been and will be. I and this race are hardly more than a grain of sand. There is nothing that compares to marching into a corral at Disneyland in matching costumes with your children. Excitement builds as the start approaches, and by the time I hear "Runners ready," I have nothing but the joy of the moment. Whatever it is, the Disney characters launching me and my daughter down Disney Way or hearing "I Love LA" blast, or someone from a charity thanking me when I really have not done anything, the time has arrived. There can be no fear and no anxiety. Time has finally passed them by, and I am free to run. Free of worry finally. My mind is in the moment. Happy to share the moment with fellow humans. Fully content.

I know this feeling at the start is one of the huge reasons I love to race. The camaraderie of thousands of people at a race all being nice to each other, all rooting for each other, all eager to do the same thing together is, I believe, literally unique in our culture. For me, the lifting of all the great emotional weights I have carried in the months leading up to that moment is joy. There is only the road ahead and the finish.

If I could live every day with the lightness and joy of race day every day, without ever carrying the unnecessary burden of worry and anxiety, I would be a happier, better person. I yearn for the starting corral.

Fear of Decisions

I have long managed my fear of the unknown with skillful avoidance. For many people, me included, making decisions can be very stressful. I enjoyed a successful career as a lawyer and executive. When my identity and sense of self-worth are not implicated, I make an excellent lawyer and decision maker. I am capable of good decisions, keep my attention proportionate to the matter, and act. For things where my sense of self or value is on the line, the simple need to make certain decisions is terrible. I avoid those choices, stressing all the time over what to do, even when there is no downside to any choice or the right choice is clear. By running from decisions altogether, even necessary decisions, I can be seized by fear of failure and as a result often chose anxiety and delay over living my life, ignoring all the opportunities for joy and learning my relatively privileged existence has to offer.

Anxiety over Decisions with Only Positive Outcomes

I was fortunate enough to get into several very good law schools—Stanford, Harvard, Columbia, and Yale among others. For weeks I agonized over what to do. Even after I made a decision to go to Harvard, sending in my card accepting admission, I could not let go. I could not bring myself to send in the card to the other schools declining their offers. I just could not. Sending in my card declining admission made my decision, a decision actually already made by accepting at the other school, more final, more irrevocable, and this was too much for me to handle. Every few weeks, I got a letter from a law school I was declining asking about my status, threatening to drop me off the accepted list, and ultimately dropping me off the accepted list. Each letter, each thought of the situation raised bile to the back of my throat, literally, not a metaphor. And this was a no-lose situation! I was ruining my life with stress created over how to split hairs among very good things. I had to pick between a bag of gold and a bag of diamonds, and I still racked myself over the choice, irrationally delaying things, even when reality had passed them by and made them, objectively, a nonissue. I could not let myself believe I had decided, even when I had decided.

My anxiety was not over a feared result or making a bad decision. There was no bad decision. My anxiety was really over the need to make a decision without facts clearly pushing me one way or another. The fact that I could not make a compelling argument to do only one thing was paralyzing. I needed an ace and had my pick of the aces of hearts, spades, diamonds, and clubs. This was terrible. If I had only one ace, I would have been ecstatic. This has to be a definition of dysfunction. To need one thing and end up paralyzed because you have four things.

Anxiety over Obvious Decisions

In other matters, I had stress simply over being the one responsible for a decision even where the decision was a nondecision; the decision itself was doing what clearly had to be done. As an adult, terminating employees, directly or indirectly, has been a source of anguish. I would put it off and off and off, even at a real cost to the business, other people in the company, and my own gut as my stress led to constant stomach pain and digestive problems. The delay was often a hit to morale of all the people doing a good, honest job and treating each other with respect. I never feared revolt or blowback. The peers of the person might be the ones demanding action long before I would consider or recommend it to my boss or client.

There is always the valid concern for the person losing a job. These colleagues tended to be young, single people with highly marketable skills anyway, who likely had offers a phone call away if not already sitting on their desk. There would be no hungry widows and orphans. That was not the source of my stress.

There was never a question about the necessity of doing it. My anguish was anxiety over the decision even though practically, it was a non-decision. I understood at the time that my delay had real costs for people, including whoever was getting fired, but my anxiety was that great.

I never wanted to be the person to pull the string that made the blade fall or, as was usually the case, the adviser who recommended it or "signed off" as a legal matter, even though it was my job to do so. Still I dragged my feet.

I had to be pushed, then found reasons to stall, imaginary reasons. I had to have more and more meetings about severance and legal exposure and everything else, all stalls over something that should happen and the sooner the better for everyone's sake. Yet I told myself one more call or meeting or memo or something was necessary before I could act or tell my boss or client that I recommended or would not advise against action.

This was not needing more time to think. I wanted to maintain the fiction that I had not made any decision or had no part in it and that there were reasons to wait. The reasons were fantasies, made-up stalls.

Whether things are known or unknown, the core of the stress is avoidance of reality.

None of This Is Helpful, Pleasurable, or Necessary

For me, the negative emotions rooted in fear are an ever-present challenge—self-hatred, revisiting mistakes big and small, decisions that passed by wealth, decisions that lost my house, prior jobs, even some lingering adolescent insecurity around sex and physical appearance. These are comfortable places. Every conversation has insecurities and self-hatred cloaked in funny self-deprecation. These are internal problems that can run ad infinitum without actually inducing or changing anything in the real world. It is just self-torment.

The fear, the stress, and even the physical consequences had to be comfortable or useful for me. Really, they *were* me, and the anxiety grew as I feared the future would take it away from me. Comfortable torment.

Stepping outside my experience, I can only assume that the long-standing social and racial hatred and false grievances of the powerful that run through our culture must be comfortable in the same way anxiety over academic and professional performance was for me. I was driven by self-hatred where other people need something or someone to hate. People like me wreck their lives with anxiety over not being good enough. Other people wreck their lives with anger at others.

It is clear that however comfortable anxiety, fear, and anger may be, to whatever extent we may have deployed them in our lives, they are not pleasant. They are not joy. They are not contentment. They are negative and painful. They are also unnecessary.

As Thoreau devised and Gandhi and Martin Luther King Jr. demonstrated on a global scale, you can effect positive change because something is right. Positive change occurs because people pursue the path that is wise and correct, not because they fear the future, are angry at an adversary, and fight.

The Dalai Lama was once asked in a recorded question-and-answer session about an instance when the Chinese police ransacked a monastery and seriously wounded fellow monks in front of him. What did he do? Wasn't he enraged? Didn't he want to fight on seeing his home pillaged and his friends knocked on the head? He explained that no, he was not angry. He did not punch anyone even in defense. His concern ran to the Chinese policemen who were doing such terrible things. He tried to explain to the policemen that what they were doing was unwise and destructive to them. He told them they would not be happy with their actions.

Is this just the nonsense a person has to say to maintain his public status as a saint? No. I think it is tactically and strategically sound for the cause at hand and personally lifesaving for the Dalai Lama. Strategically, the Dalai Lama is advocating solely for the truth. With that path, a man in a loin cloth can bend the British Empire, not to the strength of the leader or his army, but to the truth he advocates. Tactically, which is more likely to convert a Chinese policeman to his cause, a well-placed concern for his well-being and the harm he will suffer or a monk taking a pointless swing at a security officer wielding a gun? Monks taking on Chinese security forces are unlikely to succeed, even for a moment. On top of this, any violence by them would justify the aggressive acts of the policemen. Rather than feeling a burden of guilt, he will sleep well knowing that he acted in self-defense against secretly violent people. Personally how long can one burn with rage, and what is the wisdom of the decisions that would flow from rage? If the Dalai Lama indulged in anger and fought a policeman, he would be dead or rotting in a prison. If he were motivated by personal animus and rage, he would have destroyed himself, not selling books and expanding his cause decades later. Anger is not a necessity, nor is fear, nor is anxiety.

Anger, fear, and anxiety are monsters that we create . . . and we can slay them.

CHAPTER 7

Acceptance Is the Universal Antidote

You must think and act in the world as it is. Operating in a fantasy world necessarily leads only to pain and failure.

Unconditional, unequivocal acceptance of present reality is the antidote for fear, anger, and anxiety.

Such fundamental acceptance of pain diminishes pain. Pain shrinks further and instantly with thought, decision, and action.

The antidote for fear, anger, anxiety, and other negative emotions and motives is simple, but potentially very difficult—accept present reality.[13]

---

13. I understand that for many people, fear, anxiety, anger, and other negative emotions have psychiatric, hormonal, and other components. I know it is not a matter of "willing" oneself to be better, particularly without medical help. What is a tweak for some may be a herculean or impossible task for others. It may, in fact, be impossible by virtue of our physical makeup. What I am writing pertains primarily to people who generate their own anxiety and other feelings in the absence of hormonal, medical, and other external factors. Even for those whose negative emotions have a physical component, my primitive understanding, at

Face the Facts, Make a Decision, and Move Forward

Fear, anxiety, and anger are born out of a desire to be in some other world, a fantasy world where things are not as they are and where you know everything you want to know, including the future. Whether we are angry because things are not as we would like them to be or fearful because we do not know what is going to happen in the future or anxious because we want to know what cannot be known, the antidote is accepting present reality.

This is simple, but hardly easy.

See the World as It Is and Act

One of the primary therapies for clinical anxiety is desensitization. Put differently, the cure for being afraid of something is to confront that thing in real life. The solution is to move from the internal world of fears and anxieties to reality, a world where the fears and anxieties are usually unfounded or manageable. Seeing reality, the person can release their impeding emotions. If someone is afraid of cats, gradual exposure to cats leads to seeing that cats are nothing to fear. Seeing real cats is the way to chase away the fearful cats in the mind. Seeing and accepting reality is the tonic.

Accepting things as they are *does not mean* that everything is great and there are no hard decisions that need to be made, nor does it mean that you should not try to improve the future. It does not make

---

least with respect to fear and anxiety, is that for some conditions, improvement may be possible with work, as with desensitization, CBT, and other therapies. As someone with a neurodegenerative disease, I understand that there are physical limitations of each brain, and the limitations of some brains manifest themselves as fear, anger, or other states usually referred to as mood. For me, I can practice breathing, work with an occupational therapist, and bay at the moon, and the tremor in my hand will continue. Perhaps, with work, there is a controllable component or a possibility to modify my brain, but if it does not put more dopamine in my brain, I will continue to have a problem. Please do not read anything I write as "Just buck up and be like everyone else." If I am writing it, assume it pertains solely to things within someone's reasonable control or aspects of our mind that can be rewired with training.

anything better. You will still have the same injury. You still will not know if you will lose your job or finish the race. All the questions that need to be answered may still be there.

Accepting reality *does mean* that you can move forward without compounding the difficulties of the situation with the negative emotions of fear, anger, and anxiety. It means you do not need to amplify your physical pain with these emotions. If you see and accept the situation as it is, there is little room for fear, anger, and anxiety to play. Whatever decisions you make, whatever actions you take, will be rooted in the reality as it exists in the world and not a fantasy created by prevailing emotions that exist only in your head.

End the fantasy. Live in the real world.

Living each moment asking, "What is happening? What should I do next?" not only avoids fear, anger, and anxiety but in doing so makes life easier and better. Accepting reality puts the decisions you need to make in the real world. As such, it leads to clearer and more appropriate choices; greater ease in discerning the right one; picking the right one more often; and, with all of it, better outcomes.

Where fear, anger, and anxiety lead to misdirection and destruction, staying grounded in reality puts one on a virtuous cycle of easier and better decisions, each good decision creating a better reality and, with it, reducing the things about which one could be anxious, angry, or fearful.

Decisions Are Easier and Better When Made in the Present Reality

Keeping focus on the present reality makes decisions easier by limiting options to the possible—a smaller universe of options and one in which the best choice is often clear. It simplifies the situation and the paths forward. Decisions that are impossible in the context of what happens six months from now are easier in the context of the next six hours. There usually are very few options as to what you could actually do next, and very often the best choice is clear. Run, rest, or quit. The focus on the present makes the decisions required clearer and makes those decisions easier. Keeping focus on the present hacks off all the variables and scenarios running inside one's head, and it bypasses negative emotion as the driving force.

Accepting and working in present reality not only makes decisions easier but it increases the likelihood that the decisions will be good ones. Any decision shaped by or made to salve negative emotions is unlikely to help achieve a real-world goal. You are playing to a fantasy, an imaginary audience that exists in your head, not making a real-world decision to achieve a real-world goal. Good emotions and actions flow from good emotions and actions. Continuing in the fantasy of bad emotions and likely bad decisions flowing therefrom digs the negative hole you are in deeper.

Phobic and anxious people might believe things that are patently, demonstrably untrue, and these beliefs may be the strongest guides in their lives. Someone might believe that if they leave the house, they will be attacked by wolves. Someone else may have a sense that something terrible will happen, perhaps a car will hit them, if they do not touch the couch three times before they leave. It is easy to see how making any decisions based on these misconceptions, playing to these fears, would be divorced from reality. If they made a good decision about when to leave the house, it would be blind luck. Most people would claim to harbor no such fantasies. We would say that is crazy stuff and we are not crazy. Yet almost everybody does. The fantasies are just so common that we do not see them.

Nobody will ever marry me; everyone at work hates me; nobody at school likes me; the world is a terrible, hostile place; I am unloved; I am unlovable—these are common beliefs. Go to any group therapy setting, and you will hear statements like this coming from people who seem quite unremarkable. In most cases, these beliefs are demonstrably untrue. Making decisions based upon any of these fantasies is as misdirected and potentially destructive as deciding not to leave the house because you think a plane might fall from the sky and kill you. In fact, the knock-on decisions you make based on such manifest fictions could be more destructive than the original fear, because traveling in that internal fantasy world may cause you to make poor decisions at work or with the people you love, cut off people who might love you, and so on. Making decisions in the world of your dark fantasy can only bring you further and further into dark fantasy. Decisions detached from reality will almost certainly be bad decisions. Bad decisions make the situation worse. Anxiety, anger, and fear increase at the worsening situation, leading to more decisions based on a negative fantasy. The process continues, cycling toward a worse and worse reality and an internal world of greater and greater anxiety, fear, or anger. The process can dig a trench so deep into the negative and false internal world that escape is effectively impossible.

Accepting reality functions in the exact opposite direction. Accepting reality makes decisions easier by limiting options to what is possible—a smaller universe of options and one in which the best choice is often clear.

It makes decisions better because they are rooted in reality, not rumination. Good decisions lead to good results. The cycle repeats, and there is less and less about which to worry.

If we focus on the world not as it is but as we would like it to be, we are dwelling in a pointless, counterfactual fantasy. Facts are stubborn things. You will not get to the finish line if you proceed from delusional assumptions.

Cut off your fear, anger, and anxiety. Live outside your fears. Live where things are actually happening.

CHAPTER 8

Physical Pain Is Different

Pain differs from fear. Clearly seeing the causes of our pain does not end our pain. You can, however, reduce pain by seeing clearly and accepting reality.

Paradoxically, our need for pain to end increases pain and magnifies its place in our lives.

The unpalatable reality we must accept therefore is that our life includes suffering.

A radical acceptance of suffering in your life decreases pain and creates mental space for other things outside pain.

Embracing pain is difficult, but it offers the most solid foundation for hope and a better life.

Pain Limits and Destroys

Physical pain, the actual screaming and aching pain of the body, the pain of disease, decay, and injury is different from psychic pain.

Physical pain is terrible, universal, and it springs from an external physical reality we cannot control.

If we are fortunate enough to live long, we will experience pain, and pain may be the defining feature of our lives. When it hurts to walk, eventually the pain will be too great to justify walking. Walking stops. Life is then so limited. Pain presents us with the most profound problems. What is the point of life in the face of pain? What sense does it make to exist when the defining feature of your existence, all that really happens moment to moment, is pain, possibly ceaseless, grinding pain from which there can be no distraction?

I have crumbling and shifting vertebrae. The channels on the side of vertebrae out of which the major nerves sprout from the spinal cord are collapsing, pinching those major nerves, causing ceaseless pain. My spine is always moving from something that was straightish toward a grotesque curve that stretches and grinds nerves between vertebrae like millstones. I have also had cysts on the spinal cord that increase pressure within the vertebrae, which also causes pain without end short of pills and sleep. At some points, ten yards was the farthest I could walk before pain won. This all sounds terrible, a misfortune, a tragedy. It feels terrible and has been the dominant defining feature of my life moment to moment, but it is all very common. There is nothing aberrant about my experience. From a medical perspective, it is all ho-hum, run-of-the-mill stuff. A life with this pain is commonplace as, I am sure, life with pain springing from dozens and dozens of predictable diseases and accidents.

My neighbor had pain emanating from his back as well. You could see it in his face, hear it in his voice. Sometimes we would swap tales, commiserate, talking over the hedge. I have had surgeries that brought instantaneous, significant relief. These procedures reduced pain enough that other things could enter my life. One day, I was sharing my good news, trying to encourage him to hold on tight. Finding the right treatment for me was serendipitous and happened only after going through numerous doctors. Serendipity did not strike soon enough for him. He drove his car through a barrier and off a cliff. Firefighters found the car four hundred feet from the barrier—dramatic, terrible. He left a teenage daughter only weeks before her high school graduation. Horrible. I do not view his presumed suicide with any moral judgment, only humility and gratitude that I found the right treatment before pain overcame me, and sorrow for him. What my neighbor did makes perfect sense to me.

I know what pain is and how difficult it can be. I know that most likely greater challenges lie ahead, and those challenges likely culminate in death. My story, my neighbor's story, and, whether you know it or not, your story will quite likely be a tale about how to keep going in the presence of pain. There will be growing daily struggles—how to give your attention to others and respond politely, how to be productive as your prior livelihood is impossible, what to do when movement becomes limited. At some point, the pain may win out, and those who loved you at your funeral will feel gratitude that your ordeal is over. That will not be tragic bad luck. That is the way it tends to happen. Barring a real tragedy that cuts your life short, you will have pain.

Minimizing pain, therefore, holds the promise of a life worth living through disease, decay, and injury and perhaps enjoying your last day, going out with a smile on a pillow versus driving a car off a cliff. Most of what I have written deals with finding contentment amid distraction and disillusion. Minimizing pain deals with making life tolerable, continuing life when life itself is a source of suffering. There is no more important topic.

Unfortunately, I admit the insight and observations I have offered thus far seem off the mark or, at best, thin gruel in the face of physical pain. Everything changes in the presence of pain. Seeing clearly what is happening may be impossible when pain is present. If your hand is touching hot metal, the flesh burns; there is little inside a person other than the need to pull away, to cradle and examine the seared flesh, to make the pain end. Objective, dispassionate observation is difficult to impossible.

Likewise, knowledge, even if acquired, seems far from a complete solution to pain. Knowing what is happening effectively dispatches our complex, negative emotions. The anger, fear, or anxiety afflicting us usually rests on fictions that can be dispelled, and the emotions themselves are ephemeral creations of the mind that can be uncreated by the mind in the absence of mental illness. This is not to say that it is easy and does not take disciplined effort or is even possible for someone with a mental illness that impedes the operation of the mind. It is merely to say that we sense that we have some agency over these emotions, and as soon as we recognize their cause objectively, we can achieve some mastery over them.

When confronted with physical pain, knowing what is happening is not enough to root yourself in and accommodate the present reality, because the present reality is unacceptable on a gritty, physical, fundamental level. Knowing is not enough because knowing does not make the cancer in your stomach disappear or your shattered pelvis knit back together. You did not put the cancer in your stomach with your view of the world, nor can you remove it by changing your view. The cancer, the crushed nerve, the shattered bone, the disease eating away at your nerves and organs, the torn spinal cord, the destruction of your lungs—you did not make these things in the world you create with your mind, and you cannot therefore unmake them. They are part of an external reality beyond your control, and they cause pain. Indeed, in periods of intense pain, bamboo-under-the-fingernails, shattered-bone-protruding-through-the-skin pain, having great control over thoughts is unrealistic. There is only pain and what seem like hard-wired physical reactions to it.

All my philosophy seems to break down.

Pain Can Be Minimized

Despite all the unique physical and emotional challenges of pain, you can reduce your pain with thought. This was my revelation in the Chicago Marathon. This is what has transformed my life, put me on a path of inquiry, and led me to write these words. I would have said this is wholly unbelievable if I had not experienced it so clearly.

You can minimize pain.

Pain can be reduced radically and instantly with simple thoughts.

Understand this in its most literal sense. *You can reduce your pain.*

I am not talking about some broad, loose idea of mental pain, depression, or ennui to be lifted by a more grounded attitude. This is not rich LA, strip-mall yoga wisdom. I am talking about actual, physical pain, the hammer-smashing-your-thumb kind of pain.

Most of the things I have written about deal with happiness in a broad or subtle sense, ways of seeing and doing things that are wise, with benefits that may accrue in the moment or over decades. This is different. This is like having a strong narcotic pumped into an artery. It does not require learning, meditation, or anything other than a shift in mindset.

The experience of this instant freedom from much of the unpleasantness and limitations of pain was life changing for me. There are many things I have learned in the process of trying to get my carcass over the finish line. However, the lifting of pain and the doors it opened to performance and joy at the Chicago Marathon was a very personal, radical experience that sent me on this quest for understanding that has carried over into how I manage persistent, disabling pain. It did indeed feel miraculous, unlike anything I had previously experienced or thought possible. It was so jarring and its potential to improve life was so potent I had to understand it and share the remarkable news with anyone who would listen.[14]

Please validate everything for yourself, but I urge you to undertake the exercise. I am confident you will find that a turn of thought can drastically decrease your pain. This will have profound, beneficial consequences in your life.

None of this is easy. That necessary turn of mind may come at a great cost you are unable or unwilling to pay, but the possibility to reduce pain exists.

---

14. Depending on where you live and the crowd in which you travel, there will be ready explanations at hand—a god or fate or Santa or good karma or mojo or "nature." In my prior home in Tennessee, people in my shoes might wax on about the power of Christ in their heart and sign letters with a paean to Jesus "In Him." (I always found that sign-off a little creepy, especially coming from a male peer. "In Him"? Is it really better than "Sincerely"?) Here, in my native LA, people might talk about being grounded in nature or opening awareness to positive energy, terms ripped from the philosophies that created them and ported directly to yoga studios across the Westside. I once attended a yoga studio with a big sticker of the Buddha on the wall. The peppy yoga instructor would regularly say, "Look toward the Buddha and feel the burn." (Maybe the wisdom of this storefront Buddha offers the promise of rock-hard abs in just six weeks.) To me, these are lazy, fanciful explanations, yet I had this experience I could not write off as delusion.

Embracing Pain

My philosophy holds true. The general problem when facing physical pain is the same as it is with everything else, that is, a misapprehension or refusal to see and accept things as they are. The misapprehension is more subtle and the forces working against acknowledging reality are more profound when it comes to pain, but it is possible to achieve a clear view. This is a tough road, but the possibility of minimizing pain is the ultimate reward for framing life properly in the present reality.

It is true that there is a physical, external reality that the person suffering may not be able to influence. You cannot think the cancer out of your brain or heal your broken leg through talk therapy. The persistent pain that has limited my life has mechanical causes and mechanical fixes. Nothing but modifying my spine over multiple surgeries relieved pain. The problem was never a misapprehension or denial of the truth. The truth of a decaying spine was the problem.

The fact that there are real, external causes of pain not subject to thought (the fluid in the brain or bullet in the back) does not, however, mean there are no thought or emotional components to the subjective experience of pain and the role it plays in our lives. There are. While your understanding of the disease that is cannibalizing your nerve cells and causing pain may be entirely correct, your subjective experience of pain is likely exacerbated by a misapprehension of your pain as it fits into your present reality more broadly, and that can be corrected.

Much of our pain is caused by attachment to a fantasy that is very hard to abandon—the fantasy that our life should be free of pain. The cure is unpalatable and feels unnatural—a radical acceptance of pain, embracing pain as a normal part of your life.

I told you this would be difficult to accept.

Someone may appear to have a clear-eyed understanding of things. If someone asked a patient why their head hurt, they could say, "Such and such cancer cells are growing in my head and that hurts. I know exactly what is happening. I've seen the MRI. It will only grow worse, and it will kill me in three months. I will have constant and growing pain as a result." Living in contradictory dissonance with this type of knowledge is a desire to fight against the pain, the unhappiness that it is there, the belief it should stop, a belief that it is bad luck or unfair.

The person harbors a type of intimate, personal denial of the way things are. Our pernicious illusion is holding up the suffering that is our reality against the belief that we should be pain free, a fantasy. This false, persistent desire exacerbates the experience of pain and magnifies the importance of pain in our lives.

Beyond mere knowledge, a radical acceptance of the pain and its consequences is necessary. Any "fight" against it must end. Pain must be accepted as a fact, just as one would accept the sun rising. There must be a profound reconciliation with pain and the life you believe you should have.

This is a massive challenge. How can one accept what is almost by definition unacceptable? How can one not desire to be free of something inherently not just undesirable but terrible? Something so terrible that we may fall to the ground screaming when we sense it? When something really hurts, when pain is intolerable, there is a desire to hold out hope on some level that things will be or could be different, to fight against the reality even if on a conscious, intellectual level, the state of things is understood. Knowledge and understanding versus acceptance and reconciliation.

If there is a realistic likelihood that pain will pass, the tendency is to hold the days marked by pain apart as an uncomfortable purgatory, a period of life that is outside life, to support the fantasy that the absence of pain is the way things should be. We are willing to squander a lot of days to keep the days, months, and years of suffering as mulligans or rain delays and the pain-free days as the ones actually in our lives.

We want to accept pain only as an aberration, and if it must be endured for a time, on some level, it seems unfair. There is no unfairness. Pain may be part of your life. You are dwelling in harmful fantasy to the extent you chafe against the pain as something unfair or even as something you want to end, particularly when ending it is not possible. The complete truth demands acknowledging pain as part of life, perhaps even something that will grow increasingly worse, limiting ability, taking away the things you value until life is intolerable and you welcome death.

This feels like the abandonment of hope, and perhaps it is in a way. It is the abandonment of a comforting fantasy, but radical reconciliation with the fact of one's pain offers an immense benefit. Such radical acceptance reduces the subjective experience of pain. Such radical acceptance creates mental space to think about and do things apart from pain. Without profound acceptance of the pain, there is only pain and its unpleasantness. This learning and experience was a genuine epiphany for me, a miracle for a man who knows there are no miracles.

Radical acceptance of pain reduces the experience of the pain significantly and instantly. This happens in a flicker, a mere change in viewpoint and the pain is something else, something less important, a factor, but not your personality and not even your complete present experience. Radical acceptance changes the shape, meaning, and experience of pain. Acceptance turns pain from personal anguish into a circumstance to be explored and understood. It is no longer a species of personal agony. If radically accepted, if embraced, it is merely a difficult fact to manage. Unpleasant. Limiting. Grinding. Sometimes terrible, but an impediment not a tragedy.

For me, as soon as I tell myself truthfully, "This is what is happening right now; it does not matter if you don't like it; this pain is an enduring fact; this pain is what is happening; you have to deal with what is happening," everything moves. The pain abates to some extent. My thought and action shift to some extent. There is room in my mind for other thoughts not driven by the pain.

By definition, acceptance removes all the bile and fear generated by a sub-rosa denial of the fact of pain. Acceptance, forgoing the internal struggle against the presence of pain, provides the freedom to engage with the world as it is, free from the distorting lens of pain, and reap the benefits that are always available from knowing what is happening. Fear and other negative emotions lift, which, in turn, further reduces pain.

The distinction between bare knowledge and acceptance is gossamer thin and difficult to describe. It is a matter of outlook, of surrendering to the truth, no matter how distasteful it is. It is not just knowledge of facts, but how to perceive them and the weight to give them. It is letting go of any part of you that is fighting against the pain or the situation. It is making peace with the terrible and unbearable. It is a removal of intense subjective feelings and even hard-wired reactions and replacing them with what might be an extremely unpalatable reality.

If you accept reality—Yes, I hurt here; yes, the plan is off; I will not meet my expectations; those dreams are dead; I cannot walk unassisted; whatever it may be—the possibility for a better day opens. If a good day really is not possible, reality offers the promise of the best day possible under the circumstances, and this is probably much, much better than the house of horrors in one's mind.

If you accept your circumstance—no whining, no worrying, no wishing, no anger, but truly accepting the facts as facts without commentary or other involvement and then deciding what to do based on those facts—pain, not just mental anguish but physical pain from injury, decreases radically and instantly. You will still have pain. Your pain still may be too great to manage. If you could not walk before, you probably still will not be able to walk. You may still hit the morphine button as frequently as you did before. Nonetheless, your pain will be a markedly smaller factor in your life than if you compared every real moment to a parallel fantasy world in which you did not have pain.

In the standard stages of grief formulation, acceptance is the end of grief and the beginning of life beyond. Perhaps, all I have experienced and written is simply this truth in the more immediate and intense experience of physical pain. Pain and its causes are a different, more removed, less powerful beast when the self, fighting and clawing against it, is removed and replaced by a dispassionate observer dealing with a world that includes pain.

The promise is huge. Pain pegs you to one place—suffering. Acceptance allows you to retrain your focus onto positive action. Refocusing onto a positive next step also brings the promise of moving forward in the right direction, of getting off the pavement and continuing to a much happier end and a more pleasurable path.

Embrace your pain, not because it is pleasant or even tolerable, but because it is real. This is extremely hard to do, but the benefits are immense—the reduction of pain and all that follows, joy and purpose in doing things, contentment, the possibility of happiness even under very difficult circumstances.

CHAPTER 9

A Path to Minimizing Suffering

Pain is terrible, inevitable, and real.

The external causes of pain as well as the neural processes that generate sensations of pain are beyond our control.

However, our subjective experience of pain is multifaceted. The pain we feel has components we can control. We amplify pain in physical sensation and the importance we accord it with fear, anxiety, other negative emotions, and mental focus.

By changing the aspects of our subjective experience that we can control, we can reduce pain instantly and potentially greatly. This is miraculous.

Aspects of Pain We Can Control

Accepting the place of pain in our lives on a macro level radically changes our experience of pain and the control we permit it to have over our lives. We can also reduce our subjective experience of pain on a more tactical level by addressing the aspects of pain within our control.

Pain is not simple. There is a basic reaction, an autonomic physical, neurochemical response. This is not the entire story about how much we hurt, however. How we subjectively feel the pain, that is, how much it hurts and how important it is to what we are doing, has a great deal to do with our emotions and attention. Put differently, the thoughts and feelings we package around the pain and how we act in the face of pain have a great deal to do with what we subjectively feel as pain. This package we experience as pain can be broken down into three major components: physical, emotional, and focal.

The Physical Reality of Pain

There is a physical reality to pain beyond our control. If pain is caused by certain impulses going through certain circuits in the brain or the production of a chemical changing the functioning of the brain, there is an objective, measurable, physical reality to it. Your tendons stretch and tear at mile nineteen. Your stomach churns from bad clams. Real things happen that trigger some neuroelectrochemical process we experience as pain. Those physical triggers, chemical changes, electrical impulses, and many other tiny bits under our skin register as the subjective feeling of pain. If there is not a machine now, there will one day be a machine that could measure the impulses, chemical changes, brain activity, and other physical components of pain.[15]

However, even at this seemingly autonomic level of pain, the experience comes with other reactions that cannot be teased out from the unpleasant feeling of pain easily. Even in its simplest form, a collection of things cause pain, not solely neurochemical pulses caused by an injury. You hit your thumb with a hammer. You feel pain. You jerk your hand away. You hold your hand without thinking. You drop all

---

15. There may be yogic masters and the like who claim that the body can be trained to avoid or nullify pain altogether. If it is possible to will yourself to neural rewiring at a basic level, it is surely beyond the reach of almost everyone.

other thoughts to focus on your hand. There might be a seemingly autonomic impulse to crouch or flop. These reactions make sense if the purpose of the pain is to deliver a message that something is wrong: pay attention, fix it. For sure, the hammer strike begins some series of impulses, but what is triggered is more than the raw unpleasant sensation; there is action, attention, a question, and the need for answers. We package other more complex impulses and emotions around pain as well. These reactions and others are not always useful. They can be exacerbating complications. Finding a mastery over these reactions changes the subjective experience of pain.

Emotion Amplifies Pain

In addition to any base-level, physical process that one cannot avoid, there is a cognitive component to pain, a psychological and emotional component to what we feel. This emotional component is huge, perhaps the dominant component of pain in many situations. Indecision, ambiguity, and complexity increase pain. Worry increases pain. Fear increases pain.

After the scream and crouch, maybe a colorful epithet, there is a second, higher-level cognitive reaction to an injury. We hurt. We do not want it to hurt. We are angry that we hurt. We may be upset with someone else who contributed to the pain. We may be angry with ourselves. Our anger and frustration may link to other instances of loss, failure, anger, or whatever we wish. The physical pain may trigger outright anguish and despair.

A marathoner sitting on the pavement as the world runs by is likely to feel anger at the gods, the ill-fated luck that made this moment happen. It may seem grossly unfair that he is suffering pain as that guy over there is enjoying jellybeans. At the other end of the spectrum, you may be angry that getting out of bed is exquisitely painful and requires the aid of two nurses, while the world is sitting and standing and moving about as if there were nothing to it.

Whatever the physical pain may be, it is now magnified in some larger story. Dashed hopes, unmet expectations, anger, and any other negative emotion we package around pain make the subjective experience worse. It is not at all intuitive. If you asked someone why their thumb hurts and the degree to which it hurts, they would talk solely about how the hammer hit their thumb. They would likely view psychic pain, mental or emotional anguish, as a different cat altogether. Not so.

In the context of my revelatory race, pain that kept me from going another step was compounded by all my hopes and expectations for the day and how that failure sat among other failures in my life. The physical pain was in the middle of all of it. My hopes for the day were dashed. I wanted things to be the way they were in the plan and in the expectations set over months of training. I wanted to prove to myself that I was still healthy, that I could accomplish things, that I had the discipline and drive to accomplish things, and there I sat, frozen in anguish. My emotions and thoughts were inseparable from the pain. I cursed my misfortune, angry at gods in whom I did not believe. *This is not happening.* I tried to pretend. *I can keep going despite the pain if I want it badly enough.* Every thought placed the pain front and center, sprung from my fantasy world, where pain was destroying my expectations, everything I wanted and about which I cared.

I wanted the world to be the world I wanted and expected it to be, not the real one I inhabited. I wanted to know so many things I could not know. *What is wrong with me? What was my mistake? Is there some run/walk split that would make the pain go away?* I had great anxiety and fear over what would happen in the future, another unknowable. *Would I finish?*

Anguish, despair, anger, fear, anxiety, and every other useless, distracting negative emotion was packaged tightly around the physical problem. I absolutely had real physical pain. The physical breakdown and the pain it caused were real; I could not "walk it off" as a gym teacher might suggest. The pain was so great I could not run, shuffle, or walk. Maintaining consciousness was a challenge. That was physics, not a failure of will.

I was entirely in my head, reason was on vacation, letting visions of younger me, past failures, insecurities, and so on into the room. In the middle of it all was the pain. At this point, I was not really seeing, literally. The images in my head overlaid and hid whatever my eyes were actually seeing.

There was the physical reality of an underprepared runner breaking down. However, whatever autonomic thing the nervous system does to create an unpleasant feeling was magnified by the lens through which I was experiencing it. It hurt more. It became all I was, mind and body. In this state of anguish, despair, and pain all wrapped together, I was hopeless. This emotional collapse increased my pain greatly, well beyond what I felt after I had worked through the unhelpful emotional states. There was no separation between my thoughts and the pain. There was nothing outside the pain. With the elimination of the emotions and getting a beachhead in thought, I was step-by-step reclaiming parts of my being from pain and ultimately able to remediate and accommodate intractable pain to a notable extent. In the end, our subjective feeling of pain has a lot to do with the importance we give the pain in a story we are constructing in our mind. What we want has a lot to do with the pain we feel.

An Itchy Example: Desire Magnifies Pain

You can verify the mind's effect on pain easily with a simple experiment. You have an itch. Until you scratch it, it is unbearable. You feel compelled to scratch immediately, not in an hour or two or even a minute, but right now. The feeling is terrible. Even though it is not painful, you have a compelling urge to end it. You are probably a little bit out of your mind in the moment with your need to scratch immediately. Other thoughts probably leave your head, or if you try to shift your focus, the need to scratch keeps screaming to the fore.

Next time you have an itch, do not scratch. Merely observe the itch sensation with total neutrality and objectivity. The feeling is so light it is hardly there. The feeling may make you want to scratch it, but it is a much smaller, weaker thing if you observe it and see it for what it is, barely a whisper of a sensation. You can watch the itch come and go with little discomfort. It is not pleasant, but it is not terrible. There is also no great, immediate compulsion to scratch.

The desire to make the sensation go away amplifies the feeling. If you imagine your hands are tied and a fly is walking along your face, the frustration of wanting it to go away and not being able to scratch is terrible. The tiny tickle, which is all it is physically, becomes a torture.

Unmet expectation and frustration and other unhelpful emotions make the physical sensation into something much more. It is the struggle against the reality of the situation that makes the situation seem more unbearable.

A Painful Example: Detachment Reduces Pain

If you have the mental discipline, you can run the same experiment with significant physical pain whether it is a turned ankle or an upset stomach. Break out of the automatic hopping around, grimacing reaction. Notice your thoughts around the pain—disappointment, recrimination, worry, everything—and let them go. Examine your pain from a neutral, objective viewpoint. What does it actually feel like? Watch it, maybe even describe it to yourself in words. The pain is real. You will feel it. It is unpleasant, but it will be a much smaller thing. You will not hurt nearly as much. The physical component on its own, if (and this is a huge if) you can adopt a dispassionate viewpoint, is not the monster it was before. Usually, pain, even pain that was doubling-over or writhing intense, is reduced to something hugely unpleasant, but vastly smaller.

Focus Amplifies Pain

The experience of pain is stronger, more acute, and more intolerable if we train our attention on it and less if our attention is fixed elsewhere. By focusing attention and action on things other than the pain, pain diminishes. It may recede into a mere factor to be managed or diminish into an irrelevancy. It may be diluted down to a nagging distraction or, at least in moments of extreme focus, disappear altogether.

Put differently, pain shrinks if you are focused on a purpose outside your pain. If the pain is irrelevant to what one is doing, it need not be actively considered, and as a result, it actually, subjectively hurts less. If your attention is elsewhere, pain hurts less. In the simplest terms, to end pain, forget about it.

Anger, disappointment, and any other emotions we wrap around whatever is causing pain or the pain itself amplify the pain because they make the pain more important substantively. The pain or injury is front and center in the tragedy you have composed in your mind. It is the star. It matters more, and you feel it more.

In addition to the emotions in the stories we create, the very existence of the stories themselves keeps pain front and center. I can tune out a crowded city street to stew in my own hostility. Even when the world and your body are going on to other things, if you are tied up in worry or fear around your pain, experiencing pain is all you are doing and thinking. This focus actually heightens the subjective experience of the pain.

Whatever the components of our inner drama may be—a tale about an ex-wife, a bad break at the roulette wheel, the misfortune of bad health, whatever—we are focused on the pain so long as we are participating in that inner drama.

If you participate in sports, you have probably experienced the power of directing focus away from pain. You have probably finished a match or come up from a play surprised to see blood on your shirt or a divot of skin gouged out of your shins. In the moment, you felt no pain because you were completely engaged in the game. There was no room for it. You gave it no attention. The pain came after the play ended, and you turned your focus from the game to your injury.

Orange Shorts: A Real, Painful Example

An old teacher and friend later in life, my first running coach, tells a horrifying and sort of funny story: He is running a marathon. He notices that people are looking at him in horror, aghast as he passes them. He is an accomplished runner. He knows he is cruising according to plan. People are gawking at him as if he looks awful, but he really feels fine. It is a mystery. He finishes the race, happy with the result and the day. Only then does he realize that he had chaffed off the end of his penis, leaving his crotch soaked with blood to the point that blood was running down his leg. He had noticed the streaks down his leg but concluded it was the color of his new orange shorts bleeding, not his flesh.

It was a pretty serious injury. He had to spend several days without pants and underwear, waiting for the wound to begin healing. He had real pain, yet during the race, he felt absolutely nothing. He even saw evidence of the wound, but absent pain to tell him otherwise, wrote it off as a laundry problem, not an I-have-rubbed-off-the-end-of-my-penis-and-my-crotch-is-dripping-with-blood problem.[16] His focus was entirely trained on something else. Pain was not in the picture. Amazing.

One can move from painful paralysis based on real conditions to moving forward by focusing attention away from pain. It can be the difference between the inability to walk and finishing a marathon. Instantly.

Embrace Pain as a Teacher

The point of embracing pain is the alleviation of pain and achieving the greatest possible contentment while living with pain. We face cultural and social biases pushing back against our need to accept pain as part of life. Some cultural forces drive us to embrace pain for the wrong reasons. With the wrong reasons, pain will increase and contentment will be pushed further out of reach.

It is easy to say pain is not good, and it generally should be avoided.[17] However, this is not as obvious as it sounds. Our culture ties pain to ideas of success. I have been working hard to wean myself of this belief. The push-through-the-pain strategy does not work in the long term, particularly as life becomes more about managing physical decline than growth. Equating pain and success reflects unmet needs and insecurities more than any sound teaching of sports medicine,

---

16. There is also a practical lesson here about not wearing new gear for a race.
17. There are times when pain is to be expected, but you should proceed anyway. Where there is a specific intent to take some wise action that may incidentally cause pain, such as lifting weights or undergoing surgery, pain can be expected and does not signal that something unanticipated or avoidable is wrong. When you run into unexpected pain, it is generally wise to stop or slow down long enough to understand the pain. This seems obvious, but knowing this and implementing this have been difficult for me.

education, efficiency, or psychology. The experience of pain is unpleasant, sometimes excruciating. It is usually a clear sign that something is wrong. I reject the glorification of working through pain, although I am trapped in these ideas.

Embracing pain as something positive, even pursuing it as evidence of success, is deeply misguided. Pain, however, presents a positive opportunity to learn, precisely because it is difficult. Pain tests how you absorb and react to adversity. In a way, pain is the clearest form of adversity. Pain has a lot to teach us and, for this, should be embraced for what it is. If we embrace pain as something positive in itself, a sign of success, we are likely to continue down the path of misguided and injurious acts, the things causing the problems that cause the pain. If we see pain for what it is—something problematic and terrible—we can embrace it as an object of study, which, in turn, guides us to thoughts and acts that will reduce pain.

I will continue to pursue a wide variety of pleasures. Pain and its challenges, however, have vastly more to teach than pleasure. If acceptance creates space to live creatively in the face of pain, you will understand a good deal more about yourself and the world than if things come easily. Pain demands a constant examination of who you are, what the world is, and how you act within it. Passivity is not an option. Ignorance is not an option. Pain's guidance is not easy or pleasant. You are a dangling climber searching for the next handhold or the fighter trying to climb up from the canvas almost certain to receive another knockdown blow in every moment. There is virtue here as well. Our precarious existence means every day is then pregnant with opportunities to learn as one might find in the more controlled fight, climb, or race. This may not decrease pain directly, but it may give pain meaning and a defensible place in life. This relationship with pain in my experience changes the subjective flavor of pain and recasts its role in life as something that has at least some positive feature.[18]

---

18. I believe there is a sort of Heisenberg uncertainty principle for physical pain. In colloquial terms, the learning is you cannot observe something without changing it. As soon as you find the space to step back and observe pain, to crawl out of it and assess the sensations, the pain changes. In my experience, the pain decreases significantly.

I have said that running has been my teacher, but it is the pain inherent in training and the possibility of pain, of injury that gives running its potential to impart wisdom. The potential for improvement and contentment is implicit in the terrible reality of pain.

PART IV

Where Should I Go? *It Doesn't Really Matter*

CHAPTER 10

Goals

Goals are necessary to direct observations, decisions, and actions and provide motivation to move forward. The actual goal, where one is trying to go, is of no importance so long as it serves its purpose.

Trying to make a goal, its pursuit, or its achievement something more—an identity, a dream, a measure of worth, success, or anything else—is misdirection and leads to unhappiness.

Linking one's idea of success or happiness to achievement of a goal is always unwise. It places one's happiness outside one's control and will inevitably end in disillusionment.

Every life has value; therefore, every nonharmful goal is worthy.

Know Where You Want to Go

As I find so often, the real answers are more likely to be found in Wonderland than here.

> "Would you tell me, please, which way I ought to go from here?" [Alice asked.]
> "That depends a good deal on where you want to get to," said the Cat.
> "I don't much care where—" said Alice.
> "Then it doesn't matter which way you go," said the Cat.
> "—so long as I get somewhere," Alice added as an explanation.
> "Oh, you're sure to do that," said the Cat, "if you only walk long enough."
>
> —Chapter 6

The Cheshire Cat explains it all perfectly to Alice: You are Alice. You know you have to move on or remain pinioned to your unhappy spot in Wonderland. To do that, you need to go somewhere. Where? Just somewhere. Anywhere. Just not here. Is it possible you will not succeed? No. Just keep going and you will arrive.

The Cheshire Cat would likely stretch and vanish with a mocking grin as I now dive into my longer, less cryptic explication.

Quite simply, you need a destination. You have to move to live. Intentional or not, wise or stupid, moving necessarily invokes a destination.

In order to know how to make a decision, this way or that, you need to know where you want to go. Almost any direction will suffice. It is really that simple. A goal is not the defining dream, purpose, or destiny of a life. It is much less. It is a destination that shapes what direction you will go. Any nonharmful direction can produce an authentic life, grounded in reality, acting on and accomplishing real things, and producing contentment along the way.

You are Alice. You know you have to move on or be stuck in Wonderland or at least in your current unhappy spot. To do that, you need to go somewhere. To go somewhere and make decisions along the path to get there, you need a destination. That destination is your goal. Success is not achieving but moving toward that goal.

Why Is a Goal Necessary?

Without an objective providing direction, we are likely to disassociate from reality into stories that shift with our emotions. As discussed above, that is an escape from life that leads to pain. Actually living in the real world requires some kind of direction to guide what we choose to observe and what we decide to do based on our present understanding of our situation, moment to moment, day to day, year to year. You need a goal to live.

In gross terms, with no objective, you would lie in bed, staring at the ceiling. Maybe hunger and the need to pee would motivate some action. Maybe a boss or some other authority would intervene and push you around. If you were in a prison or military-type environment where a rigid schedule or sergeants made almost every decision for you, the need for an objective would be diminished. In that case, you are more along for the ride than living. You are following orders, not observing things and deciding what to do. In every decision, from the tiniest *Should I turn left or right at this point on my run? Should I continue typing or get the mail?* to the greatest *Should I get married? Should I pull the plug?* an objective is necessary. Where numerous answers are possible, you need some means to evaluate the options. When looking at the world, it is impossible to observe and remember everything. Choices are necessary there as well. You need some sense of what you need to know just to know where to look and when to pay attention.

Without your own direction, you are passive, a thing pushed and pulled by external forces. Without direction, you are a creature of appetite and emotion, unhinged desire, and disjointed experience. Your direction is whatever fuels those emotional states. You are not looking at the world and not making decisions to reach a real result in the real world. Detached from everything but the stories you tell yourself, spiraling into cycles of worry, fear, or anxiety is likely. The motivating and guiding forces spring from fantasy and reaction to fantasy, likely growing ever more disassociated from reality as the years progress. Such disconnected motivation and effort are apt to produce unhappy results. If you are wondering how your grandfather who was once a successful, reasonable man ends up a paranoid racist being fed comforting lies by television "news," this is it. You need a tick mark on your compass, or you will end up some variant of an old man yelling at clouds.

A goal is necessary only to motivate and orient behavior and make sensible decisions possible. Therefore, if the goal serves its functional purpose, neither its substance nor its achievement is important. Like Alice, it is vital to move forward to somewhere. The somewhere could be anywhere but here.

My Misguided Pursuit of "Goals"

As usual, I sit atop a mound of missed opportunities and unhappy years despite success and luxury. I am always very good at telling people what not to do. I am highly qualified to say what a goal should not be.

By external standards, I have been a goal-driven person and have semi-impressive achievements in the form of meeting those goals—degrees, jobs, titles, etc. If there was a trophy, I wanted it and would sacrifice almost everything I had to win the prize.

I wanted to get into the schools, get the degrees and marks that said even among the really smart kids, I was really good. I carried the same drive with a suicidal passion into legal practice, social encounters—everything. Everything was a competition to be won, even having lunch with someone. Without the faintest hint of a family connection, athletic talent, sympathetic story, deserving background, or anything else to put a thumb on the scales for me, I went to elite schools for college and law school. It was academic interest and drive alone that brought me to the dance. I have great stories from my high-school years, but I was miserable, verging on suicidal in my quest to win a college spot like that, all the while being considered one of the smart kids at an academically competitive high school. Stanford is the closest thing to my concept of a physical nirvana. Starfleet Academy wishes it could grow up to be Stanford one day. I have really great stories from those college years, but I was profoundly unhappy. I endured constant stress. I was not pursuing a positive end. I was working to preserve a fragile identity. In doing so, I failed to take advantage of the academic and other opportunities for improvement and discovery Stanford offered. I failed to learn from and make friends with the many creative and interesting people I met. I eschewed any idea of romantic love. In doing so, I retreated further into an idea of myself that did not require me to overcome the social insecurities that kept me from enjoying the company of others and normal life pleasures. I avoided gargantuan opportunities.

Harvard Law proved to be a great respite from this. It was the big high-school experience I never had, replete with lots and lots of vain, juvenile people, cliques, drunkenness, and what I guess is normal adolescent fun. I was semicool among the trust-fund kids and other caricatures that really do make up the Northeast elite. I was relatively fit and not a sad library creature walking behind Olympians, struggling to maintain a place by being extra funny or witty as I was at Stanford. Tradition and restaffing the inherited establishment of the DOJ and hoary old New York law firms versus irreverence and creating a better future, the former demands far less risk and creativity. Only effort is required. It is the Old World, not Silicon Valley. After all, we had all self-selected not to unravel the secrets of the brain, heal the sick, or make life easier for anyone, but to become lawyers. It was vastly easier, less stressful. The range of choices offered was limited, and the path to perceived success was as structured as a fraternity rush with employers hosting mixers and interviews in every hotel as set forth on a published schedule. I followed the path, and the path had virtues. I did not need to invent anything, bring water to a village, or do anything else that might draw an invitation to give a TED Talk. I had to study, get grades, interview, and not be as loathsome as the other guys interviewing.

Harvard was a vacation, socially speaking. It was fun and, relatively speaking, easy. Harvard Square was great. I loved being in a sort of urban environment with a subway and places one could walk. I spent afternoons at Café Algiers in a nook with a pot of tea, at the Brattle Theatre filling in my education in film, stops at Newbury Comics, the five-dollar lunch at Uno Pizzeria, the antiquarian bookseller who would give me things that did not sell, and generally enjoying the town. Even writing about it, it seems like I had it all and the gleaming bright future of a Harvard Law graduate ahead—a title, money, and status without risk or creativity.

Yet I was miserable much of the time. I came close to suicide— in hindsight, frighteningly close. I carried stress in my stomach as a near-constant pain, much of the time holding back hyperventilation. I wanted to be viewed as smart. I regularly tabulated my GPA to the hundredth of a point to determine where I was on the scale of no honors, cum laude, magna cum laude (what I wanted), and summa cum laude (all but impossible). A lot had to break my way in the final semester. I thought getting the gold star was out of reach, but I did get the magna cum laude honors that had tied my bowels in knots for three years thanks to an unexpected A+ or two in the final moments before the buzzer.

What did all the stress and bile, which rises even as I write, get me? It gave me a great start, but school brand and honors matter less and less professionally as the years roll on. You have an objective history showing your financial value. I have been out of the game for almost twenty years, excepting a brief, failed two-year hiatus from unemployment more than a decade ago. I'm hanging on, still trying, but hardly a blue sky of unexplored potential. You do not need the trademark on my sweatshirt as a stand-in for who I am. You can look at the life I have led, as a person with a family, as a lawyer with a certain capacity to generate revenue.

Along the way, I missed life and the rare opportunities I had because I was at these institutions and had a résumé that opened doors. I was willing to sacrifice too much. It might even be accurate to say I would sacrifice everything to achieve those goals because I discounted my health and consciously hoped each new task would kill me or at least render me so ill nobody could expect me to carry on the fight. I sacrificed for the wrong reasons. I was not pursuing a positive end. It did not make me happy. It did not guide a well-lived life. Nobody is happier because of my actions.

I was a goal-driven achiever in the ordinary sense and was always achieving, filling in a résumé that was uniformly top shelf. I was great hiring-committee fodder. I had great interview lunch banter, a canned character of a young man on the way up, chock full of japes, witticisms, and a clever backstory that would make me a useful and fun character in anyone's play. However, I do not think I was pursuing fruitful goals. I sacrificed to buttress a rickety, poorly designed, inapt sense of self daily on the verge of collapse. That is it. I would like to dress up my story, say what I would usually tell an interviewer, reporter, students, or audience, but I just cannot honestly. The story is opportunity lost to unhappiness and self-inflicted illness. The protagonist has been a collection of fears trying to create a person who was not afraid. Now, with the upward trajectory of life over, that false front has no value.

Yes, yes, I know this is cliché, right out of the paint-by-numbers portrait of an old man, but I look at these outward signs of setting and achieving goals, and my thoughts and feelings are dominated by sorrow, remorse, and regret.

This is not a new character arc. Even kick-ass warrior-king legends, standing on far greater laurels and titles, have sat in the same place. The epitaph of Edward the Black Prince reads:

> Such as thou art, sometime was I.
> Such as I am, such shalt thou be.
> I thought little on th'our of Death
> So long as I enjoyed breath.
> On earth I had great riches
> Land, houses, great treasure, horses, money, and gold.
> But now a wretched captive am I,
> Deep in the ground, lo here I lie.

He required the inscription to be placed at eye level so passersby could read it. This is what he wanted to say to anyone he could for eternity. The last lingering message of a grand life. I remembered seeing the quote in my youth and tucked it away as something cool enough to retain. It is no longer of purely dramatic or academic interest.

I have clear ideas and hard experience about what a goal should *not* be.

CHAPTER 11

What Is Not a Goal

I may not be able to say, for you, what the right goal is. What will define the best path, the most meaningful, and the one you will follow rests on a lot that only you can know. What direction to travel depends on subjective matters of psychology and desire. As explained above, I am a learned expert on what a goal is not.

A Goal Is Not a Dream

The concept of goals has a very big place in our culture. As the typical triumph-over-adversity story has it, a person identifies a big dream, keeps their eyes on the prize, and then experiences glorious victory. You believe, you train in montage form dragging logs through Siberia with Rocky, chasing chickens with Apollo, and you will knock out Ivan Drago in a bloody display of American superiority. Here, the concept of a goal is conflated with the concept of a dream. Dream it. Do it. Reach for the stars. A goal is a burning passion that fuels heroic action. It is outward looking, ambitious, even grandiose. It is the brainwashing I received in school that I must add something meaningful to the world, meaningful on a societal or global scale or, for the underachiever, just saving a few hundred worthy lives somehow. This is the underpinning of the Jackie Robinson quote with which I wrestle, "A life is not important except in the impact it has on other lives." On this view, a goal is something that makes a lot of people stand up and clap. This is high drama, but probably not a useful road map for most people.

In the business and self-help realms, goals feature front and center. Your prospective employer asks where you want to be in five years. Your guidance counselor asks what you would do if you had ten million dollars. Cultish religious and self-help figures, as well as mainstream business gurus, often premise everything on defining goals. Here, a goal is purpose. Without it, any justification for existence falls short. This formulation attempts to answer *Why am I here?* with an outward-looking, usually grandiose destiny. Everyone is dashing off to disrupt markets, transform lives, and turn their own life into an engine of such change.

This actually came up directly in my life as a business organizations professor. For a business organization, establishing goals as long-term planning tools is an essential task. A corporation or other business entity is an artificial person created by people for a purpose. That purpose must be clearly defined, or the entity has no reason to exist. Before the idea of a specific goal can even enter the picture, however, there must be a mission.

For human beings, I do not think this corporate outlook is particularly helpful, wise, or ethical. We are born into a life. We do not pitch a mission statement to exist. I do not think we need to create ourselves again to justify our existence. We are intrinsically, inherently a part of the world and need no more rationale than does a tree. Creating a business plan for one's life and then seeking to execute it is not a practical way to live, nor is it likely to bring happiness detached from achievement. Business plans seek to identify and exploit an opportunity. Nothing about that exercise applies to a human life.

A Goal Is Not a Quest to Maintain an Identity

My experience teaches me—actually, it screams at me—that a goal is not the same thing as something you need to achieve to maintain a sense of self. A healthy goal leads to creativity, growing knowledge of the world and oneself. Efforts to create facts that bolster a story you tell yourself or others about who you are do quite the opposite. In one, the goal is a destination. In the other, it is frantic, anxious work to give credence to a lie. One leads to growth. One tries to uphold something that is not otherwise sustained and true. One leads toward curiosity and learning. One leans toward a narcissism and grandiosity resting atop poorly contained fear and self-loathing. Working hard to achieve something you need to achieve to be happy with yourself is inherently misguided. It will produce a life of unhappiness and missed opportunities.

If you live honestly and authentically, making the best decisions you can at any moment in pursuit of a wise objective, your chosen direction, the facts you create are a product of who you are and what you are doing. They flow as a consequence from your life. You do not need to push for them. You do not have to live in fear that they may not come to be. They will be what they will be. Achievements will follow without stress or misdirected effort.

If you begin with the premise "I am a great runner. That is who I am to myself and those around me," you are sunk from the outset. You have tied your identity not to what you choose to do, giving yourself leave to adapt, but in a set, preordained identity of "runner." There is a big difference in substance, even if not in semantics, between "I am someone who is running now" and "I am a runner." In one you are engaging in an activity. In the other you have to engage in the activity to maintain your status as a runner.

This distinction is not hairsplitting. It has cost me surgeries, years of physical pain, and existential angst that has caused unnecessary physical harm and loss of precious time to misery. Most, including myself, would consider being a "runner" a positive identity. It was something of a literal lifesaver for me, moving me from suicide and illness to contentment, direction, and health, quite literally. "Runner" was the badge I wore. I never thought I was good by objective metrics, but it was what I did, who I was, my answer to the question "What do you do?" What is a runner who cannot run? Who may never run again? Who may have no realistic path to running again? The clash of the identity "runner" with physical reality—the stark, see-it-in-the-tests, see-it-in-lack-of-function, see-it-in-every-unavoidable-plain-unhappy-reality—makes every action to preserve the identity "runner" misguided and quite often destructive. If one maintains the identity "I am a runner" and cannot run, as I did for several years, surgeries, depression, pain, and the choices of addiction or suicide as solutions result. Being a runner and running are radically different things, difference as bold as pain and ease, health and decay, years and death. "I am a runner" does not have the flexibility to adapt to reality. "I am running now" does.

I think this need to identify with an activity is why there are so many lawyers. It was never a part of anything I taught, but my farewell speech to my law students was probably the only thing of real value I imparted. It was a presentation on how miserable, dysfunctional, and destructive lawyers are to themselves and those around them. The rates of divorce, suicide, drug use, and practically every other metric for an unhappy life are higher, usually multiples higher, for lawyers than for the average person. Why? Lawyers are necessarily highly educated, usually highly compensated, and are accorded status greater than the norm. My general theory is that many, probably most, law students do not go to law school because they want to be lawyers, or because becoming a lawyer is a necessary stop along the path they are pursuing. They go to law school because they do not know what they want to do. People around them tell them law school is flexible. You can do anything with a law degree. This is not so. Law school leads to becoming a lawyer. The students never knew what lawyers do, and they never wanted that life or public identity. Yet inexorably as becoming a 3L shades into the bar and then a job, the students who went to law school because they did not know what to do suddenly find themselves with an extremely challenging professional life in a profession that tags them with a lot of preconceptions and biases, an assumed place. They have an identity as a lawyer they never wanted, and being a lawyer in almost any field is an extraordinarily difficult, stressful job. They are not someone in a job they do not like. They are a person they do not like and never wanted to be: a lawyer.

Most of the successful litigators I have known do not like litigating. They feel the stress, fatigue, personal attacks, and everything else in the job keenly. They persist in it to fill some insecurity or get back at the kids who bullied them as a child. Litigating is a battlefield of dysfunction. Viewed another way, why would someone pay someone else fifteen hundred dollars per hour to make a phone call they could make or lead a negotiation they could lead? They would only need a lawyer to manage the legal arcanum that would inform the conversation. They pay because that call and negotiation are so unpleasant the client is willing to pay someone else to do it. The lawyer's exorbitant hourly rates are a measure of just how unpleasant that phone call or meeting is. That is the life of many lawyers—long days of phone calls, letters, filings, and court appearances that are painful, often hostile, often absorbing abuse, unfair challenges to their personal ethics. I have known some unflappable people who genuinely enjoy the process, viewing it all as an interesting intellectual exercise, a complex game, but not a lot of people can maintain that objective, removed repose when people are writing and saying nasty things about them in the context of usually long, complex, tedious work that mushrooms, often for years on end, with no conclusion in sight and only for the purpose of making money for someone else, a someone who themselves may be a very bad actor and in the end may refuse to pay you. In short, the world is full of lawyers who never wanted to be lawyers or do the work of lawyers. They are, therefore, miserable. The persistence and success of many in the profession is a manifestation of personal dysfunction.

The same analysis can apply to any other preordained identity. "I am a student," "baker," or even "parent." Instead of doing what you want to do, you are doing what your identity requires.

There is another equally pernicious element to approaching life not just as a specific thing, say a runner, but as a specific species, usually a positive variant of that thing, say a "a great runner." The word *great* implies some kind of exalted accomplishment or achievement impressive to others. Now you not only have to run, you have to win. If you do not, your identity falls apart, and you are left in an empty purgatory of personality. Success on the course or track no longer flows as a consequence of doing what you want to do. You have to win. That is immense stress. Every race and training cycle is a metaphysical doomsday. If you like running, this will sap the joy out of it. If you never wanted to be a runner but ended up with this identity anyway due to the expectations of others, your life is extremely unhappy. Instead of stepping out into a run to enjoy the sun and your body, to relax while working, to be happy, the run becomes a race for survival. There is a tiger chasing you, and the cost of not running fast enough is the death of the identity you have built and buttressed in thousands of other stressful runs or, even worse, the identity your parents or someone else needs you to have. Surviving one run or even ten harrowing chases is not enough. You must continually smear yourself in antelope blood and run in front of the tiger to keep your status as a "great runner." It is no way to live, particularly when such a slight change in the formulation flips the script completely. Simply be someone who genuinely wants to run and runs, if that is your bent, instead of being "a runner" let alone "a great runner."

In summary, if you are following your path, pursuing your objective, you will generate facts that reflect what you are doing and where you are going. Who you are will manifest itself in the world. You do not need to worry about achieving something or making the world stand up and clap. You do not need to do something you do not want to do, and you do not need to excel at it. You do not need the world to be something other than it is.

If your identity is being the person who can achieve something—be a great student or a great runner or, even worse, the top student or league champion—your identity to yourself and others is an artifice. Your life is a forced march to bring into the world evidence of something you are not. This is difficult. It obscures and denies what you want to do and, with it, an authentic, accurate personality. It is a recipe for unhappiness. You are both Gatsby and the party attendee he wishes to dazzle with empty display.

Check out the lawyer statistics. For many, becoming a lawyer is a path to the bottle, the pill, isolation, and the gun. It is so easy to avoid and easy to change, if and only if you are willing to alter and adapt, throw off the expectations you and others have of yourself, to be other things than what you wish to be at the moment. Put differently, the refrain again holds true here: you have to live your actual life, rooted in reality. Letting unrooted fantasies in your mind guide your life and define your identity leads to failure and suffering. A goal is a direction to pursue. A goal is not who you are.

A Goal Is Not a Measure of Success

A goal is not ultimately the measure of success or failure in life. Achievement of a goal does not even indicate whether the goal was worthy and its pursuit, i.e., your effort or your life, was useful. Outcome does not matter. Pursuit of an outcome may be necessary for the goal to function, but its achievement does not define success. In fact, chaining your idea of happiness or personal success to achievement of a goal is a recipe for disillusionment and unhappiness.

Focus on the Function, Not Completion

As discussed above, the goal itself is not important. The goal has a functional purpose. What matters is whether the goal guides your observation of the world and actions in a positive way and motivates you to keep going. The content of the goal could be writing a book on arteriovenous malformations or stacking cups. It could be free-climbing El Capitan or standing up from a chair unaided, writing a comic strip, or nuclear research.

There may be different social utility to different goals, but that, for this purpose, is only important insofar as it impacts your goal as a functional guide. Positive social purpose, that is, doing things that help people, does impact the function of a goal in good ways for most people. I am entirely certain that if decent people find the right goals for them, it will get the world to something close to optimal happiness. Every day I am discouraged by the news, but I try to adopt Anne Frank's optimistic view that people are at root good. If they are not, we, our planet, and life on it are all ultimately doomed.

Achievement Cannot Be Too Important

As a matter of logic, if the content of the goal does not matter, its achievement cannot matter. Put differently, let the Cheshire Cat be your navigator. If it does not matter in which direction you are driving or what you consider your destination, it cannot matter too much if you get to the end of that drive. There are many potential drives whose ends are equally valid. The important thing is picking the right road.

Continuing with car analogies, if you have a car (you), let's make it a dream car with amazing potential to do everything you could possibly want to do with a car. It is the Mach 5, the Batmobile, and James Bond's submarine Lotus all in one. If you are given one week with nothing else to do but to enjoy it, with no expectation of ever having a car again (life and mortality), what do you do with the car? Does it matter whether the car takes you to Pacoima or Puente, a functional trip that moves you, that you could have just as easily made on a train or bus or Southwest Airlines for seventy-nine dollars? No, what matters is the road on which you drive the car, and there are lots of great drives from the Road to Hana to the Nürburgring to bashing through the conveniently placed wall of empty boxes and fruit carts à la *The Dukes of Hazzard* and every 1970s car movie. No. You want to get the most out of the car, have the most fun with the car, do the most good with the car's unique powers, or whatever else you want. The Mach 5 has a robotic homing pigeon in it. There is a button on the steering wheel that extends buzz saws from under the bumper. How badass is that? You won't get to play with that sitting at home or taking public transportation. You want the best experience with the car as possible.

This Is Not What the World Tells Us

Whether it is the 1980 Miracle on Ice or *Alice in Wonderland* (one of my all-time favorite books sadly tainted by the apparent pedophiliac motivations of the author), the point of the story, what makes it exciting, suspenseful, and engaging is the need to achieve the goal. Achieving the goal is the concluding triumph. Mike Eruzione and company were a ragtag bunch of kids (always ragtag and *ragtag* used only in this context) who fought the Russian Goliath. Nobody thought it could be done, but we believed in them because they believed in the power of American exceptionalism, and by the powers of Jesus's love for the arrangement of our economy over theirs, those kids prevailed. They won for all of us. They had to. In novels, movies, and the stories we tell ourselves about the world, there are problems looking for solutions. There are people looking to triumph over people and nature and themselves. It is all conflict and resolution.

The stories we see in movies, read in books, and hear from

motivational speakers are about fulfilling dreams, getting to where you want to go, triumph over adversity, getting the girl, winning (especially if they say it could not be done), and so on. It is all about accomplishing a goal, reaching a destination. Even if it is a biography, all of which follow the same actual pattern of birth and then death, they insert one of these storylines. Hollywood would never make a movie that just shows the course of a life. Whether it really existed as an objective or, more likely, was just one of life's lumps and bumps, the script has to seize on a goal, a place the character needs to go.

What I am presenting is a radically different approach and one that is a little hard to grasp because we are so conditioned by Romantic notions of struggle and triumph. It is the core of drama, and we think success requires drama, when it is quite the opposite.

The real goal for Alice is not getting to the stated end, i.e., back home or catching the White Rabbit. The real goal is having a worthwhile journey. We love *Alice in Wonderland* for the magic acid trip through Wonderland. The stated goals are important only insofar as they drive Alice forward. Whether she goes this way, that way, up, down, back, or over yonder really does not matter. The rabbit is necessary as something that pulls her forward. Actually catching him would be the end. And then what? Alice would be like the dog chasing a car. What does the dog do if it ever catches the car? Nothing. It is an end, a loss of future opportunity and an unsatisfactory consummation to the quest, an exit. We should not construct our lives to view our brief time in Wonderland as failure or even something to push through. Our time in Wonderland is what we have and must be an end in itself.

Linking Happiness to Achieving a Goal Is Foolish

Linking contentment or judgment of success in any profound, existential way to meeting a performance goal is counterproductive and almost certain to breed disappointment and disillusionment.

The most obvious problem of linking happiness to achievement of a goal is achievement of almost any goal depends on many variables beyond one's own control.

Is It Your Achievement or Your Competitors' Failure?

Our culture generally defines success as defeating or ranking among competitors. There are so many factors beyond your control in winning any game or being judged well. As with everything, your physical and mental capacity are not within your control. If your happiness rests on winning a race, your happiness, your view of life as a success or failure, will be primarily determined by who shows up to run on race day. Winning or placing is about the competition as much as or more than it is about you.

Just as achievement of a goal based in competition puts your success or failure in the hands of your competitors, achievement of a goal based on the formal judgment or more vague judgments of others puts your happiness in the hands of your judges. Achievement or failure rests on the judgment of others, something entirely outside your own purview. Your success is not about what you become and even less about the things you do. Someone else confers success upon you. Your ambition is therefore to woo others. Your success is determined by how they (whoever "they" are) feel about you—unmeasurable, undefinable, and out of your control.

The Russian judge whose score has more to do with geopolitics than the ice-skating performance she judges and the judge who is not paying attention during the routine because he desperately needs to pee stand between the performer and their life-defining success. The other guys in the office, your business competitors, your boss, some idea of those who would make you lucky in love are the gatekeepers to success in a competition to have a successful career, be liked and loved, or, as is often said with no irony, being a "successful" person.

Sports and game shows with judges and scores from *The Gong Show* to Olympic gymnastics are engaging, exciting, because they are more dramatic stand-ins for how we often view our own lives. We are striving to reach that spot on the stage at that time after the performance when everyone stands up and claps. I believe we love contrived contests like this because they produce clean, understandable results from judges who can be identified and who may even provide some insight into why they judged the way they did. Attaching one's star even to the judgment of professional judges in a well-defined contest is unwise. It necessarily puts success out of one's control.

The real-world analogs for everyone who is not a performance athlete or game-show contestant are even worse. Success and failure rest in the hands of others whom you cannot even define, and the metric for achievement is often so vague there is no way to judge success or failure. Was my career "successful"? What does that mean? Who gets to tell me if it was? A neon halo does not appear over your head when you achieve fame, popularity, financial success, or anything else so you and the world knows you have succeeded. Success and failure can be defined meaningfully by oneself only, and this begs the question of why we have such a need for and definition of success. The conclusion has to be to drive a process, define a path. Otherwise, let yourself be bounded in a nutshell and consider yourself a happy king of infinite space if you get to define success for yourself. I have been around people the world would generally consider famous, rock stars even, literal rock stars, high net-worth individuals, but I have not met or worked for someone who believed they had achieved sufficient fame or wealth. They were still grasping, still climbing, always aware of the jobs they were offered or not, the money they had or not. It is simply unclear how to know when you have achieved fame, in part because the judges and criteria are undefined. It is also unclear what the goal really is. Likes? Views? Endorsements? And how many?

Is Success Determined by Your Audience?

The pursuit of fame is the dominant and destructive objective of our time. Fame is an unwise goal in the extreme. I think almost anyone would want the wealth, privilege, and ease of life that come with fame, but fame, especially pop-culture fame for being famous devoid of any activity for which one is famous, is a particularly poor goal.

Fame as a goal simply for the sake of being famous, that is, fame abstracted from any skill or attribute, just being famous, someone who cannot be described as an athlete, actor, or astronaut but merely as a "personality" is a popular and particularly destructive quest. Seeking approval from a vaguely defined population not for doing any particular thing well other than garnering the approval of others is somewhere near the height of foolishness. It has all the problems of a vague goal resting on the approval of others. Beyond this, it takes the person almost entirely out of the picture. The more abstracted from a skill or purpose the sought-after fame becomes, the less and less a person can do to achieve it. If you want to be a famous actor, you can train, work at the craft, seek employment, market yourself, get an agent and a publicist. You can try to become a famous actor by becoming a good actor and marketing yourself to obtain the desired recognition. If you simply want to be famous? Who is the judge? What are they judging? How do you know if you have won the game? What *is* the game?

Fame actually appears to be the biggest driver of fantasy and future aspirations for young people, beyond wealth, beyond being an astronaut, fireman, or anything else. Lego sponsored a Harris Poll in 2019 as part of its initiative to inspire kids to space exploration on the fiftieth anniversary of Apollo 11. Not surprisingly, Western kids do not want to be astronauts, though Chinese kids do. Among US kids eight to twelve, twenty-nine percent wanted to be a YouTuber, twenty-three percent a professional athlete, and nineteen percent a musician. Becoming a teacher did well. The only other profession in the top five—astronaut—clocked in at just eleven percent. Taken together, seventy-one percent of American kids want to be a pop-culture celebrity. They want fame. Their aspiration is having the world, not just their peers, stand up and clap. Nothing new, except the question of why they want fame. While professional athletes, music stars, and YouTubers tend to be wealthy people, wealth is not the driver here. There are other, far more realistic ways to acquire wealth—and greater wealth. In the professions kids chose, wealth follows fame. Fame comes first. So the professions chosen are the primary pop stars in the culture of this generation. (It is interesting that movie or TV star is not present at all, but YouTuber is number one.) Looking at all the professions chosen, it seems clear in the results that fame is the goal. Fame is the common denominator. The fact that YouTuber is number one by far makes it clear that fame is the goal. These kids do not want to be great pop musicians and be recognized for their ability to make popular music or be engaging pop performers. They picked pop star because it equates with fame. YouTuber, athlete, and pop star really have nothing else in common.

I do not think kids of my generation had any greater wisdom, but I do not think fame in a deracinated, detached form was the goal. It was things the fame signified and that came with fame. The goal was to be an astronaut, explorer, detective, international spy, erotic magazine publisher, daredevil in my generation; cowboy, geographic explorer, ballerina, and pirate in the prior generation. Fame was a feature and a bonus, not the end.

I want to ask the kids in the survey, Do not you dream of flying through space? Having an off-and-on-screen affair with the most beautiful movie star? Your juices do not flow when watching movies, viewing erotic material, when thinking about flying supersonic jets or basking on your own private island in some variant of a Duran Duran video? You dream of making videos that start with "Hey guys" and then proceed to an unscripted tour of your closet, walking through a video game, eating everything at a fast-food restaurant, demonstrating how to make a great smokey eye. Or, as is probably on the kids' minds, videos of a wealthy YouTuber becoming a wealthy celebrated YouTuber by showing just how great it is to be a wealthy YouTuber on YouTube.

Whose approval do you want? For what reason? How do you know when you have achieved it? What does its achievement represent for you? What does it do for you? What is your life like in the process of seeking it?

It is not clear to me why fame is the goal for so many. It strikes me as misdirected, that people want wealth, to be generally liked, and other things that are conflated with fame. As discussed above, general conditions, particularly those resting on the opinions of others, such as being liked, do not function well as goals, trying to achieve those things through the prior step of fame even less so, pursuing what could be an otherwise functional goal like learning to play music solely to achieve fame in order to achieve wealth in order to achieve a positive sense of self is misdirection on misdirection. The only purpose of a goal is to provide direction.

Goals Need to Be Rooted in Reality

The World Is Simply beyond Your Control

Even if your goal does not rest on the performance or judgment of other people, your goal resides in the world and therefore rests on the myriad variable things that can go wrong in the world. Sticking with our race-based achievement hypotheticals—time, winning, whatever—there could be a storm (or as was the case as I wrote this, a virus) that cancels the race; you could get cancer and need immediate treatment; your connecting flight to the race could be canceled and you spend race day in a motel in Denver; a cyclist could mow you down during a training run.

There is an implicit arrogance into thinking that achieving something, even something that seems entirely within your purview, is really within your purview. Whatever you are doing rests on variables and variables feeding those variables and an exponentially growing body of variables that could not be identified completely by a thousand supercomputers daisy-chained together. You do not control the world. You cannot predict or even catalog all the things that could impact you, let alone control them. You cannot address many of them with meaningful action. There are lots of things that are just one in thousands of a chance to go wrong, but there are countless thousands of those. The world is something to be navigated at best and quite often just endured.

Simply put, you do not control the world and cannot anticipate the circumstances in which you will work. (People just get sick, even die. I am told this is quite common.) Linking your happiness to achievement of something, as opposed to its pursuit, will almost certainly produce disillusionment and unhappiness.

Mistakes Are Inevitable

There is a fragility to investing in a specific result. There is often an implicit desire for things to play out exactly as imagined—no unforeseen problems, no mistakes, no external difficulties. The focus is on getting to the end, not on finding and following the best route, and this leads to errors and makes necessary course changes more difficult.

You will make mistakes. You will fail to achieve your objectives. You will do so in unexpected, unpredictable ways. You will do so in stupid, inexcusable ways. You will.

If one wants to get to the sought-after ends past the error, the best approach is one that puts focus and effort on working through that error. Linking happiness to achievement is sure to lead to unhappiness.

The Paradox of a Specific Achievement as a Goal

Strive, train, race, live to win, so long as you understand that winning is unimportant.

Trying to win a race is a fine objective if it functions as a goal. That is, if it guides decisions and motivates action for you. The point, however, is not the winning. Actually winning, achieving the goal, is unimportant. It is the work, the life lived in pursuit of the goal that matters.

Is this possible—to work, maybe orient one's entire life around winning a race, yet be disinterested in actually winning? I think so, but it runs against the grain of our cultural orientation, which tells us, as UCLA coach Red Sanders did, winning isn't everything; it's the only thing. The trick is to maintain a functional, daily view of the world while understanding that in a broader cosmic sense, even in regard to personal happiness, none of it matters.

At the risk of getting overly esoteric, this is an everyday manifestation of, at least for me, the core challenge in practical philosophies premised on the selflessness of existence. There is no self. There is no you. Look for the thinker of thoughts inside your head, and you will find no such person, no homunculus typing out the thoughts and pulling the levers that move the body. Yet there must be a someone looking, a someone engaged in the exercise of looking for that thinker of thoughts. You cannot even discuss the concept without accepting yourself as a talker and someone else as an understanding listener. Self or no self? On a practical level, both things are true: (1) there is no self, no you in any permanent, important way, and (2) your pants fit you and not another guy, so there is this thing, a you, that wears those pants, puts them on, and looks for the self that is nowhere to be found. It is a fundamental paradox. Like Captain Picard overcoming Q's conundrum to prove humans deserve to exist in the first and final episodes of *Star Trek: The Next Generation*, which is all we have, the string of episodes to death, and then there is no question that the self is not there. We must hold two contradictory notions in our heads at once. This problem sounds very Eastern Philosophies 101, but it is not merely esoterica. It filters down to the most mundane decisions and actions, like, Do I put on my running shoes or turn on the television instead?

The importance is being on a path, drawn forward toward a goal regardless of reaching the end. In designing Disneyland, Walt Disney talked about buildings as "weenies" in the experience of the Disneyland guest. Walt's dog, the story goes, would go anywhere in pursuit of a proffered hot dog, a weenie. The hot dog was a sort of force manipulating and driving the dog. In Disneyland, big landmarks like Sleeping Beauty Castle were "weenies," there to pull the patron inexorably forward to it. We need a Sleeping Beauty Castle in our lives, pulling us down Main Street and not letting us drift aimlessly or backward out under the berm into the meaningless drift of traffic on Harbor Boulevard or in our minds.

In practice, the paradox of moving somewhere and being agnostic as to whether you get there is much more easily managed in living than in the abstraction of philosophy. My goal in running is to finish or finish in a certain condition or within a certain time. My objective in form is no different from that of a runner seeking to set a world record. My prior objective of finishing a marathon in five hours is no more important than another runner in the race setting a world record. I also understand that things change. In the course of writing this, I have been given new diagnoses; my body has changed, and I have a different anticipated path. My goals must change. Finishing in five hours, finishing, running ever again, walking to the corner, writing—they are all equally valid goals and as worthy as seeking to set a world record. It is fine to strive for the finish, even for the podium. It is fine to strive for the mailbox. I can make those things my objective, and if they guide a happy life, they have served their purpose.

I can also not take any objective too seriously. I cannot take myself too seriously. Understand your place in the broader scheme of the world. Take a social or even cosmic view of who you are.

Even if the objective is more important, even if the objective is to feed five hundred hungry people that day in lieu of running, from this personal point of view, actually feeding the people is not important. Of course, whether the hungry person gets fed or not is of literally vital importance to the hungry person. However, feeding the man is not a task destined by fate or some other written rule in the universe for which you alone are responsible. It is not so even if you make it your own overt goal. Achieving that goal is not even a matter under your direct control, though it is a wonderful goal to pursue. The real purpose of the goal is to guide work with diligent focus to feed the hungry, which is also the best way to feed the most people. If anything, linking personal happiness to achieving this or that goal of feeding the hungry, believing that it is your specific mission and that your life is measured by that metric, is likely to lead either to a sense of failure or to a belief that the job is done. Either of these states discourages further effort and will not feed as many people as would ongoing, motivated, directed work to feed people, detached from any identification with success or failure of the task. Motivated work born of contentment and, as with everything, a brutally honest view of who and what you are is the way of the most ardent, constant, and successful philanthropists and generally good people in my view. Success and accolades follow joyful, motivated action. With this approach, doing good becomes a vocation, a path, not a specific prize.

It is cliché, but true. It is the running of the race that matters, not the time or place at the end. If you are directed and motivated to keep running, you are more likely to finish, get the time, or win than if you invest your sense of worth in any achievement.

It is simply unwise to link one's sense of accomplishment, worth, satisfaction, or anything else important to any actual achievement.

Life Is a Path, Not a Racetrack

At the root of it all is the fact that life goes on until death. The only positive thing there can be after the achievement of a goal is another goal. There is no finish before the grave. There is no end point, no finish line, except the grave. There is nothing etched in the universe that says you must do x or y to be happy. If you think achieving a goal is an end point, you will be disappointed. After a brief hit of misguided or at least self-induced euphoria, you will see emptiness.

At Disneyland, unlike some of the other, newer parks, the castle, here Sleeping Beauty Castle, is just a double-faced facade, effectively two-dimensional. As soon as you cross the bridge to enter the castle gate, you are exiting into another land. The castle is not really a place to be. There is not an interior where one could rest. If the purpose of your day was to reach the castle, you would be sorely disappointed. The castle is essential to the progress of your day, but in itself is nothing, merely a moment that ends as soon as it begins. It is a torii gate in fairy-tale design. The castle is a goal. Its function is to draw you down Main Street. It is the thing most identified with the Disneyland experience, despite it being totally ephemeral as a part of the experience. Once you are there, it is behind you. You have stepped from Main Street through a short tunnel to Fantasyland. You must look to a new landmark and continue to move through your day.[19]

---

19. There are claustrophobic hallways and staircases one can enter from the castle periphery, where dioramas have been displayed over the years, but the experience of being in the castle in the normal course of a day is walking through a tunnel perhaps fifteen feet long, much like the experience of walking through the gate of an actual castle or medieval college.

CHAPTER 12

Picking the Right Goal

Defining a goal that fits you and your desire to increase perception, understanding, and happiness, while also keeping you free of physical and psychological pain, is what matters.

Calibrate the goal to maximize happiness and give yourself permission to modify that goal as new information about the world and yourself is discovered and your own thinking matures.

A good goal is rooted and achievable in the real world, holds your interest over long periods, guides everyday decisions, and requires positive action.

Find the right goal, and happiness will follow.

A good goal must guide life and in doing so will give life meaning. It must be interesting enough to keep us motivated, difficult enough to keep us growing, a good-enough match with our talents to breed feelings of success. In short, it must function as a goal, an objective that directs observation, decision, and action and also keeps us marching happily down the path the goal shapes.

A Case Study in Delayed Happiness

Up until recently, I thought going to law school was the great personal tragedy that put me on a trajectory to be miserable amid apparent success and status. The source of my unhappiness was not the profession I chose. Though lawyers are a miserable lot, I have seen people find happiness in the law, and not all of them are dupes who have convinced themselves that they are really helping people. Some of them do help people. More know they are not but live happily anyway. My father enjoyed the law and did, indeed, help many people plan for their end and resolve family disputes.

My problem was not my profession, nor was it pursuing goals as opposed to more direct sybaritic pleasure. My problem was I picked the wrong goal. Academic success and soaring as a lawyer are not inherently the wrong goals. They were the wrong goals for me. I was not at all suited by personality for my profession. The person I wanted to be and who I told the world I was would have been a great lawyer and happy living as such, but that was not the actual me. The right goal for my false, almost farcical identity was not the right goal for the real me.

My life story could be framed as serial accidents of picking the wrong goal and the resultant misguided effort, disappointment, loss, and depression. In a way, I never picked a goal for myself. I did what garnered praise—from my mother, peers, institutions. I walked in the direction of conventional wisdom. I went to law school because . . . that is what you did if you were a humanities guy and smarter but less personable than the guys going to business school. Yes, I picked the path in that I filled out the applications for the schools and the jobs, but I never looked at what a lawyer is or what they do or who is happy or unhappy in that slot. Never. I never even looked at the broad stats I made sure my students understood about suicide, divorce, drug use, depression, and every other negative metric for lawyers. (For my students, usually second and third years, it was too late to turn back, but I hoped the understanding of the potential for negative results would make them more careful in their choices than I was.) I was always along for the ride with some caricature of who I wanted to be driving. Even when I hit the wall and tried to reinvent myself, what did I explore? Writing and teaching, exactly what the script called for. I never really chose and I certainly never made a wise choice about what goal I should pursue.

My misery was compounded by the engrained belief that to mean something, my work had to have real social value, that I needed to help others for my life to be valid and my work a worthwhile use of my time. This added pressure did not help matters.

I did not find a real goal, a useful objective that guided my days by the months and years as well as by the hours, keeping me moving happily through life toward positive ends, until I started running. Will I ever be a good or successful runner in a broad, objective sense? No, and I am not trying to be. Nonetheless, training for races and giving myself the reward of race day has been a productive, happy path. My running goals are the best goals I have ever had.

Your Goal Must Be Tethered to Reality

Much of the time, we are living in an internal fantasy and acting based on winning, looking good, shoving it in the face of our nemesis, going back for the third curtain call, or something else in that internal fantasy. Our facts are our own creation, and reality is window dressing. That is where most people live, I think, most of the time. Reality is in the way.

Yet we must live in the real world, however much time we spend in our minds, navigating an internal fantasy. Our lives take place in reality. We must make decisions and act constantly. Every moment, with every decision from *Should I eat this Mallomar?* to *Should I swallow the pills?*, we need something to guide our actual, real-world actions. The question is usually not whether we will stay busy. The question is whether our actions will be guided by fantasy or something real. The path of fantasy leads to increasing disconnection with reality, increasing failure and frustration as we are smacked in the face over and over again with external facts.

Anyone pursuing a goal in the storybook Hollywood—doing something grand with heroic action, fighting toward victory against all odds, leaving everyone gobsmacked who said it was impossible and our enemies on their knees begging for mercy—is almost certainly letting a fantasy guide their decisions. That certainly was the case with me—studying and working too hard, picking my profession, choosing my friends, denying myself things that made me happy was all done in furtherance of goals that lived in a world of fantasy, stories about who I was. To make it stick better, I would tell myself stories about the way the world was, but this just pulled my life choices further off the mark and made my life within the real world less and less tolerable. I spent my adult life trying to be respected and good at a profession that brought me pain, and not metaphorical pain. Every time I had to make an unpleasant phone call or just enter a normal negotiation or any other contact, my heart would race, acid would rise to the back of my throat. I would hyperventilate. Speaking would be hard. My body is reacting this way now just thinking about it. A sane person would not persist in the career for years and years when the most basic everyday tasks induced panic. It was beyond a dislike or malaise. It was physically painful, and more than once my body just quit on me altogether. Ultimately, my body made decisions for me because my conscious decisions were so destructive.

My fantasies, my stories about who I was and who everyone else was grew ever darker, deranged, and disassociated with reality to continue down my chosen path. I was being guided by a fantasy formed from graphic novels, movies, a comic-book-level reading of history, my parents' expectations, the praise of authority figures, and egotism. I would soar as a scholar, a lawyer, everything else and be recognized for doing so. I would make a difference and have everyone read about it in the paper. The goals took me to intense study of historical arcanum; a high-level, high-pressure legal career; at times, a conventional social life that did not fit; and things only got worse. I was making myself increasingly unhappy because I was making decisions in furtherance of an idea of the person I thought I should be based on fictive values and views of the world. My concepts of success never evolved much past my childhood idolatry of Batman, Captain Kirk, and Robin Hood. Indeed, that idolatry continues, only now with the masking irony of the committed geek. I would never be the person I wanted to be. If I somehow were Batman, James Kirk, and Robin Hood at the same time, I probably would still be deeply dissatisfied and consider myself a failure. My goals lived in a make-believe world and were not attainable in the real world. Not a good way to live.

Simply put, keep your goal tethered to reality with adamantine chains. If your notion of where you want to go is informed by movies, novels, or television and not by the things you currently can do in your life, you are likely off the mark.

A Goal Must Be Achievable

Corollary to keeping one's objective rooted in actual circumstance, pinned to the facts that comprise a life's environment, are the benefits to keeping the goal achievable. A goal firmly planted in the soil of reality will be achievable. It will have a defined end. A goal that cannot be achieved cannot guide human behavior in a realistic way. It could work for some purposes, but ultimately the path forward will crash into the facts that make the goal impossible.

A good objective is not an aspiration. It has to have a clearly defined end. I will eat better. I will exercise every day. I will study more. I will slow down and relax more. These are not functional goals as I am defining them. The foregoing are aspirations for general behavior. There is no success or failure or path to them. At root, they are broad, general wishes. Developing positive habits is important, but a habit is not a specific objective. A habit does not guide much behavior beyond the habit itself. Who are you? What are you seeking to achieve in life? The answer cannot be "I want to eat more leafy vegetables." A functional objective must have an end.

This may not seem like much of a limitation, and it is not. There are countless objectives one could have. However, we have a tendency to envision our future in loose dreams or attributes. I want to be famous. I want to be rich. By themselves, these are not objectives. There are innumerable paths to make those adjectives applicable to you. The adjectives themselves are loose and tough to pin down. Wanting to be rich does not on its own guide decisions. Something more specific is required, such as starting a business or becoming a doctor. When we are lost in internal fantasy, we generally do not picture ourselves doing things. We just imagine having the dream girl or car. We generally do not fantasize about the work to get there. Dreams are not enough. Life is the work to get there.

A goal could float in the hazy realm of what is currently not possible but may be impossible. This is the world of innovators. Some areas of innovation likely provide sufficient direction to guide a life. The innovation itself follows a well-worn process or ventures into things standing on other achievements that make the way forward logical. As I write, three vaccines for COVID-19 have just been validated as effective. Choosing to pursue a vaccine in a tried-and-true method or even more novel mRNA methods has a logic to it, a pathway that provides guidance. The facts bear this out. It appears every line of research and application was successful, the science meeting reality in a matter of months. Working toward such a goal makes sense even though success is not assured. It is reasonably achievable enough to guide behavior. A goal like creating an alternative to all known vaccination methods divorced from any existing methodology to follow is a dream. It does not tell you what to do when you wake up. Discovering a new, yet unimagined form of entertainment, locomotion, or anything else that does not follow from what is known and relies on serendipity is not a useful goal. You could lead your life so you are well positioned for a new, unexpected discovery, but you cannot walk in a direction totally unknown. It is not a possible direction. It is an aspiration.

I have been reading recently about how the understanding of Parkinson's disease has unfolded since James Parkinson in 1815 lumped a number of frequently coexisting symptoms into a conceptual bucket that would ultimately bear his name. From the outset, unpredictable, unexpected, blind luck accounts for much of what is known. Parkinson happened to notice similar traits among a population of patients. More than 150 years later, the link to dopamine production was discovered because several catatonic drug addicts washed up in different San Jose–area hospitals. Someone noticed that there were several patients with the same bizarre symptoms in the area, traced their commonality to use of heroin from the same batch that contained an unwanted, brain-destroying chemical known to be harmful from other research into toxins. The study of those toxins showed a link to the failure of nervous system functions reliant on dopamine. The similarity of symptoms between the drug users and Parkinson's patients provided the link to Parkinson's disease. Thus from an early nineteenth-century clinical practice to paralyzed drug users in the 1980s, we learn that insufficient dopamine is at the center of Parkinson's disease. Wow. A botched bag of designer drugs, catatonic addicts showing up in Bay Area hospitals, all linked to a neurotoxin led to the central, present understanding of Parkinson's disease and, therefore, the primary means of its treatment, that is, drugs to increase dopamine levels. This kind of discovery is super cool but not a viable goal.

Many scientists put themselves in a good position to field a ball that might be hit in their direction, but the quantum leap and new direction in understanding, here as perhaps always, is primarily a result of good fortune. You can follow leads based on existing knowledge. You can learn and place yourself in the game so, like the 1980s doctors in San Jose, you are ready to see new things and walk down the paths those new facts suggest when coupled with your existing expertise. The link with dopamine was unknown. The path from bad heroin to that understanding was entirely unpredictable. Nobody could get up every day and take steps to discover that. Catatonic addicts do not fall from the sky every day. There were doctors, however, well prepared to seize the unpredictable opportunity and set new goals deploying their expertise in new ways.

As a definitional matter, you cannot walk toward the unknown.

The Goal Must Be Achievable by You

Be honest with yourself about your present ability and play within your game.

To function as a goal guiding decision and motivating action, the goal must be achievable by you. It is not enough for something to be achievable in some abstract sense. Looking to what the laws of nature or even prior human history say is possible is not enough. It must be achievable by you in your present circumstances. It has to be realistically achievable within the bounds of practical effort within a time frame that keeps you motivated. A useful goal, therefore, rests on an honest, clear-eyed account of your present abilities and your realistic potential to improve in the time frame of the goal. In short, you need to play within your game.

This does not mean achieving a goal should be easy or not require pushing boundaries beyond what you think you can do and certainly beyond what you can do today. It does not mean that your long-term aspirations should be limited by your present ability and potential. There is a place for thinking big.

The purpose of setting realistic goals is not to define down a goal so you are certain to finish first or even finish. It is not to make sure everyone gets a trophy just for signing up. Rather, the point is to ensure that the goal exists in your world, the real world, not fantasy, because the goal has a real-world function. Your goal exists to guide your life toward a defined end. It is not the stuff of dreams. It is the stuff of what you can and should do right now.

No amount of will to do better will change certain aspects of your ability in a given moment. That is the truth of things. This view runs counter to the Disney/motivational speaker if-you-can-dream-it-you-can-do-it mentality, that nothing is impossible; you just have to believe in yourself; wish upon a star; nothing is in your way but small thinking. This is not so. Objectively. Demonstrably.

It would be foolish for me to set qualifying for Boston next year (or any year) as a goal. It is not a realistic aspiration. I have spent the last nine months just trying to get myself to a strong walk. I am old by running standards and have infirmities. My realistic, first milestone is to run again. This is not a gimme. I have been working at it through PT, surgery, and drugs, and I am not there yet.

I am nowhere near training for time, and even if I were, I would never qualify for Boston. At age sixteen, as a high-school runner sixty pounds lighter, I could not do two miles at the Boston pace. Starting with the best possible physical case for me with the aid of a time machine, qualifying for Boston would not be realistic. If my goal requires going beyond what is realistically achievable, I risk being discouraged by the impossibility of it. Qualifying for Boston as a life direction may be supported by dreaming, thinking big, just believing anything is possible if you want it badly enough, but none of these things touch reality.

My extended failures over the last eleven months are a result of the pitfall I am cautioning you, dear reader (which is me right now), to avoid. I have been holding out the goal of running again even though I cannot achieve a brisk walk. I am focused on running even though I am injuring and reinjuring myself with daily activities and even though rolling over and getting in and out of bed is a real challenge.

Because I have been thinking about things outside my present game, running or even walking well enough to finish a significant race, I have not been playing at all. This leads to inaction, atrophy, and depression, not a life moving forward toward one's full potential.

The lack of motivation to hike to failure is also a prod toward fantasy. If reality screams, "You will necessarily fail," you will have good reason to retreat into a fantasy world where negative facts are not facts, reason does not matter, and your desire is external reality. Instead of guiding you forward in life, real life, your goal will push you deeper and deeper into delusion and denial, fear, and anger.

I do hold out running again as a broad objective in a hazy future, but there are many, many things I must do to get there that are far away from running.

Most people associate goals with dreams, and dreams are delusion. My child's sixth-grade yearbook listed what each kid wants to be when they grow up. The general theme is everyone thought they would be famous. The boys' standard responses were NBA player, NFL player, or both! Some wanted to be pro lacrosse players or other things that just are not things to be achieved. Reality will drop a boulder on top of almost everyone's sixth-grade dreams. They will then have an option— accept reality or live in fantasy. They could pretend that there will be a pro lacrosse league, so they better train and be ready for that day. They could pretend that even though they did not make it through the high-school football recruiting process, if they just work hard enough, an NFL scout is sure to invite them to the combine tryout. There, they will somehow perform at an elite professional level, even though they never have come close to such ability before. The longer the fantasy continues, the more difficult acceptance becomes, and that difficulty accounts for the angry baseball dads, cheerleader moms, and others who lived in dreams until they switched to bitterness and transference to their children.

None of this is an argument against thinking big. Keep tent posts out in the distance. If I were sixteen and absolutely committed to running, qualifying for Boston one day would not be a crazy thing to think about in a misty, barely visible possible future. Even at sixteen, a decade or more of dedicated work and progress that transformed me into a radically more capable athlete would be required. I would need to make varsity long before I could make Boston. Still, I could think about it and work toward it. Today, no. So many things would have to change, including arresting or curing a degenerative neurological disorder for which there is no cure. I can work toward the dozens of major objectives along the way to becoming a competitive marathoner. Perhaps that work would change my circumstances enough to think about what may be outrageous goals today, but that is a future reality that must be created with practical goals today.

The Ethics of Pursuing Your Own Goals

Every life has validity. Every life can have purpose regardless of circumstance. Every path one chooses to pursue has potential to guide a fulfilling life of discovery, thought, and action in the world from cradle to grave. I have done lots of things that I can make sound interesting and important, but for me, they represent years wasted. I found direction and meaning in running. It served as a direction to guide a productive life of healthy action and intellectual exploration. It is an activity done infinitely better by a hamster, and I will not kid myself by saying it helps raise money or sets some example; it has no direct social value. If anything, it is a waste of my education, experience, and potential by conventional standards. My ambitions as a runner peaked in second grade when I was the second-fastest in my class and crapped out in ninth grade when I failed as a cross-country runner. I am a bad runner by external metrics and will never rise to the level of okay recreational jogger. If my objective really were to help my local food bank, it would be vastly more efficient to give money to the food bank and to devote my time directly to the cause than to sign up for a race. If I wanted to apply my knowledge and experience in law and business to feed the hungry, there are many things I could do. There is a great deal I could have done with the literally thousands of hours I have spent running and the tens of thousands of dollars I have spent in its pursuit. No. I run for me. It directs a productive, happy life, which, in turn, may lead to broader positive activity, but that is not the purpose of the objective. It is a consequence that flows from the well-adjusted, productive life inextricably tied to pursuing a realistic goal and rejecting fantasy. I am a better person and more likely to do more of value in the world, because I have given myself an objective that does less.

The graduation-speech view of goals does not lead to happy, productive lives. Rather, it leads to hunger, need, disappointment, conflict, enduring failures in pursuit of triumph. It leaves a lot of people out. The person confined to a room whose joy and vocation is keeping bonsai trees, the monk who spends his life in cloistered meditation and study of religious arcanum, and the man with nothing left but making a good fall in the face of death can lead wonderful lives as valid as MLK's. I would like to think that this is some aspect of the equality for all that MLK championed.

This smaller view of human achievement fosters medicine, engineering, and other socially useful things. People will gravitate toward these things if they are thinking clearly and seeing the world for what it is. They provide interest and positive feeling. They are wonderful playgrounds for the short life of a human. However, they are not the only ones, and from an individual's point of view, working to cure cancer may not be a better path than working to perfect card tricks or an even more isolating and less cerebral pursuit, running.

I always wanted to do something worthwhile as I was indoctrinated to desire. I often did things that looked worthwhile from the outside. It looked like I was reaching for laudable stars and catching many of them, but I knew it was all a ruse. I knew I was not helping anyone in any important way. I was an academic lawyer for a time. There is little less important in the real world than law review articles. It is an exercise of one academic lawyer writing opinions and ideas for an audience of a few other academic lawyers who write on the same subject and make their careers criticizing what their few colleagues say, a well-researched, repetitive loop of drivel. To compound the worthlessness of academic law, the discussion is almost always of a world the professor thinks ought to be, not the one that is. It is fictive writing in which no sane person could take pleasure. Historical research on the Great Cat Massacre of Paris (yes, that is a thing) promises far more value than anything I wrote, work that was probably read by fewer than a dozen people and whose relevance has been passed by actual events. Yet we think law professors do worthy things. People would ask me to speak and interview me about topics in which I was no expert because that status of university law faculty held a glamour. Often, my reaction to a call by a reporter or invitation to speak at a conference or business was "Uh, really?" Law professors play an important role in important public discourse, right? I was a law professor; ergo, I had important things to say. I was doing something worthwhile or important as evidenced by my place at the podium while the room went to work sawing through hotel ballroom chicken.

Even though my practice had a role in discovering and then settling the legal frontiers of the internet and media distribution, about as exciting as a legal career in business could be, I do not think I helped to save a life or even make a child smile. There was no real social utility beyond an argument that someone in society had to do it, and confronting this fact led to deep disappointment. (My apologies to everyone who received music or movies more easily online, but what you are doing has limited social value, and my role as your ancestral servant in the cause has less.) In my heyday, my speaker's bio made it sound like I was a legal genius and entrepreneurial maverick. I was a very good, unusually creative lawyer, but I do not think any genius I or anyone could have would manifest in law. I worked for entrepreneurial mavericks. Even if I had a maverick idea, I was a lackey. Whatever potential I had was wasted in my profession. I was unhappy because I knew this.

There were always people around me—subordinates, students, some clients—who thought sitting in my chair represented a worthy dream, an important step or end in a life lived well. At each professional stage, I soaked in this praise for a few years but ultimately found it corrosive and quit. I did nothing useful and nothing that would not have been done by others equally well. I helped the really wealthy grow really, really wealthy. I helped students advance to a career that would make most of them miserable. At best, I facilitated innovators, but it really was the innovators doing the work, and the innovators around me were not saving lives or feeding the hungry. They were trying to get movies, music, software, and information to people. My professional life had the aura of someone who must have had worthy ambitions, worked hard, and achieved them, but I knew that aura was an optical illusion. Anyone who thought otherwise just made me feel like a fraud. I could not pretend that I was doing anything worthy. I would quit, move on to the next thing that seemed like a dream role in life, to discover the same emptiness.

I was leading a goal-driven life, goal after goal, focused effort, and sacrifice, always leading to achievements that proved to be of little value and, as such, were a source of disillusionment. I had no concept of what constitutes a healthy, useful goal and what is a sentence to misery and possibly destruction. I was misled by my belief that a goal, a life path, had to be something others would deem worthy.

There is no question in my own life that the unlikely, seemingly selfish, idiosyncratic pursuit of running, not my chosen profession, has replaced anger and cynicism with gratitude. I am a better person, doing more in the world, caring more about the world and those around me, because I have given up on doing what my life directs me to do and doing what I wish to do, however inconsequential the activity itself is.

You do not need to be the best at something. You do not need to change the world for the better. You do not need to be famous. You just need to know in what direction to walk.

CHAPTER 13

How to Get There

Working is path and purpose. Moving toward goals gives the things you do meaning. The things you do are your life.

When it comes time to perform: Show up. Do not try. Drop all goals and expectations. Have fun.

Preparation over time alone defines performance. Thoughtful planning work over time is the only path forward and the only sustainable way to improve.

Stop trying. You are the runner you are on race day. The runner at the starting line is the real runner, and she is a product of thousands of miles of practice over many years. Powerful desire, grim determination, anger, and any other self-created stress do not increase your capability.

Having fun and not trying does not make you perform materially worse and leads to better decisions than determination, anger, or any other self-created stress.

These better decisions might be the difference between finishing and never starting.

Let the real you perform, as you are at any moment, doing what you are capable of doing with radical acceptance of yourself and your situation, embracing change in every moment.

Acceptance, even of disappointing facts, may open a door to performance you thought impossible under a view constricted by assumptions and expectations.

Along the way, seek expert help and avoid the Siren calls of ego, ecstasy, and distraction that can divert you from your journey. Keep the goal alive in every moment.

In absolutely everything: Stop trying. Have fun.

Another Revelatory Running Experience

My third marathon, which was also my second Los Angeles Marathon, contained confirmations of what I had seen before and some new, stark revelatory experiences about how to perform even when performance seems impossible.

I dove into my training for this race early and with great enthusiasm. I did not have to stress about finishing. That was a given. I had done it before and then done it again. The only question was how well I would do. (Oh, such unwarranted hubris and disrespect of the distance.)

In my mind, I was a runner. More than this, I thought I was a marathoner, or at least I could say the marathon was my current distance. With the stress of reaching the finish line gone, I thought I could just run worry free. Run I did, too much, too fast, too long, my desire way out in front of my physical ability. I did not pay attention to my pain. I was thinking about times, reading about strategies for getting through the aid stations, granular details about diet and how to be incrementally better in everything every day. I could live in the weeds of such minutiae because I knew I could finish. All my effort turned to being better.

In the immortal words of my people: Oy. I was the running equivalent of a freshman who believes he understood everything about human behavior and desire because he finished his first six weeks of Psych 101.

Not surprisingly, I developed pain. The biggest pain was in the center of my forefoot. It hurt with every stride, with every push off that foot. I continued to train as I wished. It just felt so good to run and to know that I could run. After all, only a few months ago, I had this amazing experience in Chicago in which I proved to myself vividly that I could finish despite really significant pain and the mental problems that flow from a physical breakdown. I continued to run as I wished with confidence. The fact that I was running every day through increasing pain just showed how hard I was trying and how capable I had become. Not surprisingly, my foot injury continued to worsen.

I ground to a halt, unable to continue running, with the race only a couple of months away. I was really in a panic. Once again, my errors in judgment and discipline were threatening to rob me of my prize, the goal, and the day in which I had invested so much hope, so much work, so much ego. My desire to succeed and my desire to do as much work as possible to succeed were the very things that would keep me from succeeding. I tried to delude myself into thinking all would be well by continuing to run, but things got worse and worse, reality trumping my fantasy, until I could not run at all. The pain in my foot was winning.

I bought many new shoes in a panic, hoping to find the equipment that would take the pain away. I was the Imelda Marcos of running shoes, cycling through more than ten different models, looking for the magic bit of kit that would save the day. That effort failed. You cannot buy your way out of a foot injury. I was not able to run.

I saw my podiatrist/serial Boston qualifier, who became something like Mick to my very poor version of Rocky. He built a rig of pads in my shoe that cradled the fractured bone off the ground. After a month and a half of healing, I was moving, in pain, but moving. All was not lost.

Race day approached. At the time, I was living in Memphis, so I made a family vacation out of the trip to Los Angeles.

A Setup for Certain Failure

I am always trying to get my family on the fitness bandwagon and, more specifically, to join me running. I convinced my wife to do the San Diego Half Marathon, which was the weekend before my big day. I was committed to her success. Running would be great for her, and somewhat selfishly, I indulged in reveries of us living out our golden years running in races around the globe. I made the decision that I would train and run the race with her no matter what.

This became a growing problem in the lead-up to my race, as training with my wife was in addition to my own marathon training schedule. Where I was and what I was trying to do just did not match up with her goals and status as a new runner, fresh off the couch. I played coach and ran by her side, spurring on my hope of this as a family vocation. The runs were slow and easy, but the extra miles on me added up and hurt. I knew this was a big factor in escalating my injury, but I did not want to let go of her success or my dreams of being in a running family, our matching outfits and costumes marking us as a happy, healthy crew. Here too, my desire and motives were good, but my decisions foolish.

We ran the San Diego Half Marathon the weekend before the LA Marathon, and we did finish, but due to my poor coaching, my wife was poorly prepared. We were on the course for close to four hours and had a long walk and wait on our feet before the race as well. I do not think any training plan suggests a 13.1-mile race a week from the real race day, but this race with my wife had immense value. I was willing to sacrifice my marathon for the hoped-for future with my wife.

The day took a much greater toll on me than I anticipated. I had some muscle soreness, and my injury announced that it was going to be a factor in every step henceforth. I was walking, but it hurt.

In addition to my overriding commitment to my wife (which was also a commitment to myself), I made a commitment to my children that I would keep even if it meant sacrificing the marathon altogether. We love Disneyland, and I promised that we would go every day during the week. Even if I had to scuttle finishing the marathon, my children would have as much Disneyland as the span of our vacation would permit. I would match them step for step, line for line, hot fudge sundae for hot fudge sundae.[20]

So following our trip to the San Diego Half Marathon, in the five days that preceded race day, I logged more than fifty miles walking in Disneyland according to my GPS watch and stood in line for dozens of hours on top of that. I was limping and physically struggling through much of it. It was joyful, but taxing. I know my children left with the memories of us at Disneyland I wanted them to have. I have no regrets, but it was unwise in the extreme, looking at things from the perspective of marathon preparation.

You Must Show Up

Woody Allen is reputed to have said, "Eighty percent of life is just showing up." I will take it further. If you do not show up, you may be hiding from your life, cutting off experience, and locking in failure because certain, voluntary failure is easier than accepting change and doing the work that is possible. It sounds stupid, and it is simple, but a

---

20. Even though we live near Disneyland and spend thirty to forty days per year there, I live by a personal Disneyland creed. I will never tell my children we have to leave. Whenever they want to get there, usually at rope drop (which means leaving at 5:00 a.m.), I go. We stay until they want to go home, usually until closing at midnight, with the ritual second dinner at In-N-Out, usually with a child asleep on the table, then the drive home to follow. Back-to-back full days means three hours of sleep or less for me as the driver. This is tough over the course of a week. However, my children will never have a memory of their father making them leave Disneyland. Never. As with my wife's half marathon, this is hardly a selfless move on my part. Every moment at Disneyland with my children is a gift for which I am grateful, both in the moment and in memory. Please bring back runDisney!

gating issue for absolutely everything is showing up. It is very easy to convince yourself that there is no point in showing up and often very hard to suit up and go, but it is essential. Perhaps showing up is eighty percent of what there is in life, but if you do not show up, you do not get that eighty percent of life, and you are not eligible for the other twenty percent either.

You have to show up.

Showing up opens the gates to experience you may not have anticipated or thought possible. As Bilbo is reputed to have said by Frodo, "It's a dangerous business . . . going out your door. You step onto the road, and if you don't keep your feet, there's no knowing where you might be swept off to."[21]

In my case, race day loomed. I sat up the night before, sore and hurt. I stuck to my priorities of my wife and children, but I did not think they would bring me this low. The marathon and all that went into it seemed lost. Going to Dodger Stadium on virtually no sleep and then running seemed like a lot of unpleasantness leading to more unpleasantness, pain, and certain failure. Would not the better course of action be to forget about the race? Be realistic about my status? Be kind to myself, remembering the wonderful days I enjoyed with my kids? Be grateful for getting another day of vacation with my family and forgo the race? That may have been wise. My reality (injury, fatigue, and pain) was entirely at odds with my desire (running a marathon). I had learned at the Chicago Marathon to be realistic, to make wise decisions based on reality and not the fantasy worlds of my own desires. That was the framework of the situation to me: reality versus desire.

Reality should triumph over fantasy, but yielding to that wisdom meant *not running*, and this went entirely against what I had invested in this moment. Here, I reverted to my accustomed motivations of self-hatred and a need to prop up a false identity. Old habits die hard. Not going was quitting. I do not quit. If I did not try, I would not have felt wise; I would have felt weak, like a coward, a failure. I could not make forgetting about the race feel right. I lay in bed, sleepless. I was

---

21.   J. R. R. Tolkien, *The Fellowship of the Ring*, The Lord of the Rings vol. 1, London, England: HarperCollins.

tormented over whether I should run, and if I did not, what it meant and how I would view myself and the months of preceding effort.

I would love to say that I made a wise choice, but I ended up with a good result by falling back on another of my engrained emotional weaknesses—indecision. I punted. I told myself I would head to the start of the race at Dodger Stadium. There, I could make the determination as to whether I could run. No matter what, it would be fun. Anyone who has run a marathon knows the singular enthusiasm of a marathon start. I deserved to be a part of that even if wounded. As an Angeleno, sitting in the shadow of Dodger Stadium; downtown LA twinkling below me; people from every neighborhood and ethnicity; the thousands of kids from Students Run LA given a life-changing opportunity, all of them joking, hopping with excitement; a beloved Dodger player whipping up the crowd; the elites straining to hear the shot go off; I could enjoy all that. I was not a poseur. I logged the hundreds of miles to get there. I was just hurt, even if due to my own often foolish decisions, but I could give myself that hard-earned cookie. I could at least sit and watch. These were my thoughts as I lay in bed.

At 3:00 a.m., not having slept at all, I got out of bed to start my big day. As soon as my feet hit the freezing tile floor in my parents' house, I stumbled forward. The pain was unexpected. I had to put on my shoe with the funky rig to make it to the bathroom. This was absolute idiocy. I would not even make it from the Dodger Stadium parking lot to the starting area.

Still, I suited up and went. My body would loosen up enough to walk, and I would enjoy the day however I could enjoy it. This self-talk seemed like pure fantasy. I drove to the race. I was probably the tenth car in. I am always nervous, so I arrive hours early. At the LA Marathon, this provides a unique opportunity to walk around the stadium before the crowds arrive.

I was sitting in a nearly silent fog in front of Dodger Stadium, for me, the pantheon, the font of all things noble and blue. I was looking up at a multistory-tall portrait of Jackie Robinson. Jackie, who he was and what he did, is a living presence in my home. Though he is from a prior generation, as a dad, he is the go-to example and aspiration for so many things, ethical, physical, political.

I knew I wanted to run. *What the fuck is wrong with me? To think of not even entering the corral?* Of course, my thoughts also ran to our greatest Jew since Moses, Einstein, and Groucho—Sandy Koufax. If Sandy could pitch two shutout games with only two days' rest in the World Series with his wounded arm, I could at least crawl to the starting line. *Maybe Sandy will emerge from the stadium in Dodger blue Jedi robes and say the Hebrew priestly blessing over my foot.* I was truly moved at being in a place of such beauty that has such meaning in my life, the shrine of Jackie and Sandy before me, the once active workplace of Tommy, Garvey, and Cey and then Hershiser and Gibson. Was all this intentional cranking up of emotion with nostalgia and comic-book plotlines the right motivation? No. Not at all. It was all rooted in fantasy, fantasies about baseball and heroes, fantasies about who I was and my situation. I was fortunate in that this motivation was extremely powerful motivation and really, just by luck, drove me in a positive direction.

I wanted to run. I knew that much.

Applying Lessons Learned

Assess My Situation

I did not go forward with blind emotion. I remembered and applied what I had learned, notwithstanding the tears that were already coursing down my face. I examined myself closely, honestly, as I had learned to do in Chicago. I assessed my body, the physical reality. It was going to hurt, but I was not going to cause permanent damage to anything if I walked or even tried to run. I had faith that the rig in my shoe would keep any fracture from expanding beyond the point of healing at some future point. Even if this little nugget of bone in my foot shattered into one hundred pieces, there had to be an appliance or screws or something that could keep me walking through life.

Reframe the Problem to Meet Reality

I thought about what was really going on. My difficulties that morning were not a necessary product of my injury. The crack in my foot and the pain were real. The difficulties, however, were self-imposed, a product of viewing things with the wrong frame of reference. I was assessing the situation relative to the objective of finishing and not finishing. I was clinging to fantasies of how I would perform from a place of total hubris a year earlier.

Trying to get any corner of reality to line up with that template of success—finishing the marathon as hoped—was folly. That template projected failure from every angle on the present reality. Meeting those preordained expectations of finishing the marathon and maybe even doing it in style were not the only aspirations one could have.

I could give myself the opportunity to have whatever experience I could have. I did not need to lock in the failure of not seeing where the journey might lead just because I would not meet the maximal hopes formed months ago under an entirely different set of facts.

I could not run a marathon. Thinking about crushing 26.2 miles was absurd. I could not run well for even one mile. I could, however, run some distance, probably walk even more, and I could make it one of the best days of my life with the right approach. I knew this at the time. This was a conscious understanding and choice. Happiness was a choice. I just had to let myself enjoy the day. That meant letting go of my prior goal.

By abandoning any concept of failure for the day, failure itself became impossible. If I jettisoned all hope for a specific performance, by what standard could I fail? Only the abandonment of prior expectations and desires let me enter the corral and opened the possibility for happiness.

As in Chicago, I made a pivotal decision that changed everything, only here my objective was pared back from "I'm going to finish" to "I'm going to start." I deserved that, the thrill, the high fives with strangers, "I Love LA" blasting from every speaker and not for a baseball victory but for me and everyone around me. Wow! Would that ever happen again in my life? That anthem. Playing there. For me and all my race-day brothers and sisters. I would give myself that, and I would stretch out as much distance as I could with the sole goal of having fun.

I really did not know what would happen. I was very confident I could run across the starting line and probably walk the first few hundred yards at the stadium, maybe even make it to my beloved Disney

Concert Hall—Dodger Stadium, Disneyland, and Disney Hall in a one-day period was heaven for me, places I love. If I could, I should let myself have that, not struggle through pain in anguish to reach some arbitrary goal, but let myself have it through whatever effort I could make.

I was in my corral, back with the steerage, the runners playing for a dream more than a time. I was going to "run." I was with my peers, my best friends for the moment, high-fiving, wishing everyone the best day ever, hugging strangers, feeling absolute joy, everyone infused with the exuberance of a life peak, thousands of people for one day sharing a common goal, kids literally jumping with too much energy to contain, oldish runners like me playing for their own triumph, a cross section of the wonderful smiling people of LA, gallons of adrenaline and dopamine flowing through the crowd, each drop a contagion for another drop in someone else. There are not many people fiddling with their watches or warming up in corral K. There are a lot of people amped with gratitude for reaching that day, so many, at least for the day, giving the finger to cancer, a rough home or school life, addiction, and low self-esteem. I had already given myself a gift by letting myself be there. I had earned my place in that corral. Once I was there, any thoughts about not starting, about not running, were gone, as gone as the option to lie on the pavement in Chicago was. There was no fucking way. I would make this my race, whatever that may be. This was my race. My day. Already, I was having and would *continue to have* a great day. I was going to run, maybe not out of the parking lot, but I was going to run.

My decision was made easier because the matter was different and bigger than finishing the race. It was a decision to be part of whatever beautiful social moment was happening. Downtown lay below, Hollywood and beyond to the ocean to the west. I could almost feel that first zephyr of cool ocean air that shows up at mile twenty-five to let you know the finish is near. Jackie looked down with approval as I went over the timing strip. It was not just my personal triumph. I was surrounded by smiling, cheering friends, all of us with different reasons for doing the same very hard thing together. I never felt such love for strangers. I genuinely wished a perfect day for them. I never would have made it to the start if I were alone and not one small part of something much larger.

How did I move from self-hatred, failure, and paralysis to active joy so rapidly? Reality did not change. My thinking changed. Why did my thinking change? I am not sure. It was a voice of greater wisdom in my head that rose above the self-pity and pain and demanded to be heard. The voice just arose. I may have nurtured it, given it the script through months of preparation, but I did not conjure it. That voice of reason, called mindfulness or "wise mind" in popular parlance, that little mental shift turned what may have stood out in my life as a year of failure into a worthwhile year climaxing in one of my best days ever.

How did I follow this new path? It was a radical departure from the hundreds of hours of planning and preparation I put into the day. I was able to follow this path not because I had achieved great discipline and enlightenment, but because no other path was possible. My new framework presented a Hobson's choice—run without expectations or don't run.

My pain, injury, and difficulty were a gift in a way. They led me to the abandonment of expectations, and this, in turn, made everything a source of new gratitude and joy. I was not going to even start. Now I would. Every little bit of the day was its own victory. By effectively turning off my watch, prior or present expectations, my day would be measured by the enjoyment I would have. With every moment being a gift, this had to be a magnificent day.

Forget about Your Goals and Don't Try

A plan that puts no pressure on your performance enhances performance and makes for a great day.

The evolution of my plans: Plan 1. Stay at home; Plan 2. Show up and watch; Plan 3. Cross the starting line. That's it. After that, I would not try to do anything with the race. I would make no effort.

I really did it. I really did not make anything like complete effort at all. As a result, the yards, then miles slipped by. I finished the race. Repeat, **I [full stop] finished [full stop] the bloody marathon!!!!**

Vin Scully's call of the famous Kirk Gibson home run was in my mind: "In a year that has been so improbable, the impossible has happened." I was living the impossible.

In the course of one day, I made the journey from too hurt to go to the bathroom without my special shoe to turning out 26.2. The key—I really did not care about finishing. I really did not try. So I finished. I did not care. I did not try. Therefore, I succeeded. No kidding.

I walked every uphill segment. I stopped when I wanted to. Took pictures. Peed. Made phone calls. Tied my shoes many times to get my feet as comfortable as they could be. I walked when I wanted to walk even if I had the energy to run. I let my mood and body determine how I moved. I was pursuing happiness.

Whatever I was doing, however comfortable I made myself, I was always moving. The hours and miles started to pass. I talked with a lot of people. As usual given my sloth-like pace, I was back with the firefighters and soldiers in full kit, middle-aged runners like me proudly flagging that they had cancer a year ago and were there crushing LA that day, oddballs committed to dancing the whole way, lots of different people with different stories that I was happy to hear. I was happy to share my own. I was living an impossible gift, and I knew it every moment.

Maybe Thomas Jefferson was my true running guide. I had forgotten about running a race and was simply enjoying the liberty I had given myself to pursue my happiness. This, in turn, permitted me first to start, then not push to do more than was fun and therefore finish the race.

My foot injury was not a significant factor. The thing that hurt that morning and about which I had been obsessing for weeks, spending a fortune on equipment, medicine, and anything else I could do to manage the pain and anxiety—it just was not a problem. Yes, the pain was there, always there. It hurt a lot and made itself quite known in every step, but I was able to move. I did not collapse in agony. I was able to talk. It was a constant, like a jackhammer outside your office window. I could let it be the only thing in my life or a background hum tuned out by keeping my focus on other things. The pain went from being an unconquerable challenge to a background nuisance as I had experienced in Chicago.

The day was a lovely, slow, unhurried odyssey. I snaked through Chinatown and Downtown, Silver Lake, Hollywood Boulevard, Beverly Hills, Century City, every mile reminding me of old friends, old apartments, old jobs, and the places a younger me and present me liked to be. This is my home. Walking let me enjoy places I have driven through a thousand times with an emphasis on driving through. Not driving or even running, but walking these neighborhoods for the first time, I got to meet people in Little El Salvador, Filipinotown, Thai Town, and elsewhere, accepting the treats and high fives the children offered. These neighborhoods were filled with warm, smiling people. The LA Marathon may be a nuisance for the denizens of Beverly Hills. In other neighborhoods, it is a wonderful, welcome big deal, and the people, kids, grandparents, everyone wants to welcome you with oranges, treats, funny signs, even chili dogs. The course is a tour of my life, the stage where my life has played out. Walking so much without any regard for time or how far to go let me live the course in a different way. If there was a kid who offered a high five, I took it. If there was an old lady offering candy, I took that too and the gift opportunity to exchange smiles with someone I otherwise would not have met. I had the time, and that was not a diversion. That is what I was doing.

It was an unforeseeably great day, different than I had planned and worked toward for so many months, but certainly better.

Trying Hard Can Turn a Great Day into Misery

I was really enjoying myself and was amazingly fresh up to about mile twenty-one. It was unreal. I was far more at ease and energetic than I was during my long training runs. It was easy and fun. The pain was now just a part of me, really unpleasant but not in the way. I had a lot left in the metaphorical tank, having taken it easy all day. Because I felt so great, because I felt as fresh as if I had just been out for maybe eight miles, not twenty-one at that point, I decided to try really hard the last five miles. A mistake.

I gave all I had. I ran as hard as my body would permit, and I was really unhappy during this effort. The race went from a lark, hanging out with various crazies on the route and loving every yard of LA into a grim trial of pushing through pain and multiplying failures of my body. Those miles were substantially faster, much faster, maybe ninety seconds per mile faster than my average miles, and that speed burst is at the end of a marathon. However, the cost was very high in terms of effort, pain, and recovery time. Trying to do well was a mistake. I should have stayed with fun. The reintroduction of aspiration and effort was unwise, a stain of misery on an otherwise perfect day.

Trying Hard Does Not Really Increase Performance

You are the runner you are on race day. If by natural ability and training you are a runner who turns out twelve-minute miles, that is the runner at the starting line, a guy who runs twelve-minute miles. There is nothing you can do on race-day morning to change this. Going materially faster, if possible, would be a product of months of training and diet. The thing you are doing is the thing you are doing. Trying extra super-duper hard with anger and desire that exceeds practical ability really cannot move the needle too much. It cannot change your real identity, which is the product of preparation, the life you have led, not your feelings as you wait for the gun to start the pack.

My discovery of this was a real surprise. After making it across the line, screaming and crying in triumph, doing my best Muhammad Ali victory pose for the camera, I looked at my watch. I was in disbelief. I really thought my battery quit or I had hit pause accidentally. In the end, I finished with almost exactly the same overall time as in my other marathons. Craig not trying with an injury was a little slower than Craig trying very hard and suffering, but not a lot slower. My overall effort of twenty-one miles not caring and five miles of really trying and hurting myself was almost identical to trying hard the whole time without an injury. It seems impossible. How could flitting and hobbling around, taking photos, talking with people and just not trying or caring produce such a time? It did. Interestingly, the injury was not a factor.

In the end, the difference between hours of misery and hours of fun probably amounted to no more than 7 minutes out of a 345-minute run.

In any race, when balancing effort and ease, I could

1. Have fun. Take it easy the whole way and just be a little slower.
2. Take it easy most of the way and use whatever energy I have in a burst at the end. The combined time would be roughly my time trying hard the whole time.
3. Try hard the whole time, be miserable the whole time, and end up with a substantially similar time to the times in the prior options. Faster, but not so much faster that you would care unless you were running for time.

This spectrum of options does not present a difficult choice.

The difference between truly not trying—walking whenever running seemed hard or just not fun, taking time to talk to people and express gratitude, calling my kids—and grinding out the miles in misery was just not that significant. I am the runner I am. The runner I was on that day was birthed and shaped by biology, diet, and, most important, months of training. Trying harder or not on race day does not change the physical realities. I could not "will" my way into being someone else with a better mix of attributes and training.

This was revelatory, that my final time after hanging out, walking up the hills, and otherwise going on a five-hour frolic was not much slower than grinding out the miles through a haze of pain with grim determination. Not trying is about the same as trying. Amazing. Does this mean I am really fast? Really slow? Well prepared? Not prepared? I don't think it means any of those things. I think it just means I move my body through 26.2 miles about as fast as my body can move through 26.2 miles. At any given moment, I am the runner that I am. Improvements based on effort are marginal.

As Yoda put it, "Try not. Do or do not. There is no try." You are the person you are doing the task you are doing. I can see no difference between just doing and really trying beyond the minor physical changes we impose on ourselves with trying. I do not think trying does anything beyond adding a tightness in the stomach and jaw during the effort. Doing and trying. Waiting and enduring. What is the difference? I see nothing but the insertion of ego into an otherwise factual situation and the introduction of physical stresses that are almost certainly unhelpful.

If you want to perform differently, live a different life or pick a different activity. You are the person doing what you are doing. You do whatever you are doing as well as you are capable of doing it.

There is no destination in real terms. It is a concept, ephemera, created and uncreated as a mere idea, some flash of neurons with no impact on the world beyond the chemical soup of your brain. This too is another rephrasing of the tripartite paradoxical box of truths—you need to pursue an objective, the objective does not matter, and achieving it does not matter. Your happiness and meaning must be walking the path toward the objective. All other ideas are built on fantasy and will almost certainly lead to unhappiness. Embrace the practice because it is actually the game.

Embrace Change

Embracing change is vital, and it needs to be more than just a willingness to modify things when confronted with error. It needs to be an attitude, an approach, a way to work, live, and succeed.

As circumstances change, even the best-fitting objective and best plan to get there must change. Something that was right a week ago may not be right now. The plan also may have been wrong a week ago. Clinging to the old plan in either case is putting ego and fantasy over reality. Reality will win. Whatever the cause of the change, even if it is due to one's own failure, that is the past, and the present is reality. Adjust and move forward. All else is a pointless competition between what is and a fantasy of how you wanted things to be.

This brings us back to the importance and necessity of spotting and acceding to change in the context of the fundamental paradigm—what is happening/what should I do next. In order to see what is happening, truly, actually happening, to see things as they are, devoid of our own ego, desires, and fantasies, we have to be completely open to change. To see clearly, we have to be an iconoclast with ourselves as the icon to be smashed—our most treasured, self-defining beliefs being the most important things to smash.

Seeing things as they are lets you set an objective and make a plan to get there based on reality. As you walk your path, observing with a keen eye and an open mind, new facts come in, circumstances change, you change. For your goal to serve as a functional goal, you may need to change it. Your most productive and enjoyable means of getting there may change as your understanding of you and the world changes.

As with so much in here, there is a hint of paradox. To get to where you want to go, you need to change where you are going. It is a shadow cast by the general truth that your objective tells you where to go, but your objective and where you end up do not matter. I am not terribly bothered by this. I am writing what I have observed to be true. If there is a flaw, it is less likely to be the truth of what is asserted than ignorance of how disparate truths connect.

This is true: without an openness to change, contentment is likely out of reach.

Because I am resisting changing my own goal around running, I am unlikely to have a fruitful life. Because I am resisting changing the means of getting there, I am extinguishing hope and replacing it with despair.

Knowing and doing are such different things. I believe I will change on both counts—goal and methodology. I will just waste a chunk of life grieving for the impossible.

PART V

Happiness

CHAPTER 14

Is Happiness a Choice?

Happiness Is the End

Happiness, however defined, has to be the beginning, end, and purpose of our journey, what we seek and what we wish to maximize along the way. Happiness is the currency of life. We could play semantic games. What about the masochist for whom pain is pleasure? What about Cameron, Ferris Bueller's gloomy friend who was only happy when he was sick? If we demand happiness fit some narrow filter of experience, like physical pleasure versus physical pain, these are problematic questions. Not here. Happiness is the end sought.[22]

What composes happiness? It can be almost anything, as it is solely a matter of perspective and personal desire in the absence of unmanageable pain and privation. As pornography was to Justice Potter Stewart, I think happiness is to the well-functioning person—they know it when they see it. Not so for me during much of my life and I am sure many others like me, but happiness is what is sought.

---

22. Even if every person may define their own happiness, everything I have written suggests some forms of happiness are wise, others not.

Thus far, almost everything written deals with minimizing pain, dispelling fears, rejecting fantasies, and continuing through challenges to results believed impossible. Much written has a pessimist's perspective—how to soar above the storm, not how to navigate only in the sunshine. Alleviation of fear, anxiety, pain, and anything else in life's pandemonium is a sort of happiness, or at a minimum, its elimination makes space for joy. The outlook and process I describe is a path to a sublime equanimity, a happiness beyond the normal pleasures of satisfying a (typically delusional) desire or the implicit pleasure of avoiding pain. Everything I have written, however, is a great deal of work and mucking about through one's mind and circumstance. It is easy to understand but difficult to impossible to do. Does one really need to do all this thinking, observation, and disciplined effort over years, making each moment an event, likely through trials of pain and fear to get to happiness? Maybe not.

There are happy people. If you have a handle on what happiness is for you, why not just be happy? Forget all I have written, just listen to Bobby McFerrin's "Don't Worry Be Happy." Is that possible? Can you simply choose to be happy and be happy?

My Father: Happiness Is a Choice

Several years ago, my father and I went on a trip together to Yellowstone in Wyoming. This was not at all a typical thing for us. We were not close. He had health problems. I had some health uncertainty. I lived a thousand plus miles away. This seemed like a good thing to do. We could have some time together, in effect, to say hello, get reacquainted, and then say goodbye, with no regrets that we did not spend any time together when there was time. The trip was a life highlight.

My father was better than a great person. He was a decent person, an extreme rarity. He maybe gets a C on the Jackie Robinson standard of measuring your life in how you positively impact others. He took the easy way whenever given a choice. He never learned about how or took any steps to enhance his compassion. He never worked on managing his anger (there wasn't any) or other negative traits (I don't know what they would be) to be better for others.

He was just a decent person. I am sure I have run across others, but I cannot think of any. Everything he did, even if limited, was generally good. When he did good, he did not know he was doing good. He was just being his comfortable self, doing the natural, obvious, easy thing in his situation. He did not need years of meditation practice to achieve this postwar, comfy equanimity. He naturally helped everyone in his orbit, expected nothing in return, never used his magnanimity to bolster his ego or tear down the recipient of his help. He was befuddled when he was thanked. He did not overtly give. He was not a volunteer. He was not a philanthropist. He was not in the donor class. He never sought to make a big positive splash in the world, just live a happy family life by the standards of the 1960s middle class. (Jackie is shaking his head that someone born with so many material, educational, and social gifts squandered them on merely being a nice guy in his community while the country was in the throes of the civil rights movement, Vietnam, a cultural revolution, and so many other things.) He was simply balanced and good natured through and through wherever he was, whoever was around. He was that person always, and being that person, he helped those around him without ever trying or thinking that he was helping. He was a rock, not in a spartan, tough-guy way. He was completely comfortable in his own skin all the time. I cannot really imagine him any way except at ease, happy to have gravity hold him in his chair, a mug of gin in his hand, and an open expression on his face (or sleeping). I have never seen him run or even hurry. Really. Even when we played catch as a kid, he would saunter to a missed ball, to my great frustration. He has had ups and downs for sure—he was treated very unfairly at work; his professional standing and experience were vanished in a changing economy; he faced unemployment, kids with drug, social, and mental problems—but it never got to him. I can recall a handful of moments, truly fewer than five, when he was emotionally distraught, one of them being the death of his father.

He liked life. He did not want to be unplugged from any machine under any circumstances. He wanted every second of life possible. To him, it is a good world, and he had no desire to leave it, regardless of whatever adversity and pain he has faced and may face again. This left us with little to say to each other. I just looked at him with some envy. I'd like to be in his world. I live in a different one.

This is the man with whom I traveled to Yellowstone. I did have an agenda. I wanted to find out what he wanted from me when his time got short. I also wanted to tell him what I wanted from him when sickness and death were at my door. At the time, it seemed very possible that I would predecease him.

We sat in some well-themed steakhouse near the park, with a stone hearth, lots of exposed timber, maybe some antlers here and there, and I raised the topics. He wanted nothing from me. He just wanted to live no matter what, under all circumstances. Illness, pain, and death are nothing to get in the way of anything. No surprise. I knew this. What I wanted to communicate to him is I am not like him, and for those reasons, he needs to stay far away and keep the rest of our family far away if I need to manage my pain or my end while he is still alive. I knew we were not cut from the same cloth and my choices would seem misguided and self-destructive.

He understood and reminded me that he had already lived this scenario. He reminded me that his father killed himself. I had forgotten because the manner of his death was a nonevent to me. I did not know how that suicide hurt my father. My grandfather: Old. Alone. Terribly alone. Generally unwanted. Invited to family functions out of obligation. Not fun. Not warm. His business sold ten years earlier. His wife dead for several years. Handicapped and unable to go places on his own. It seems like ample cause to say goodbye, and in functional terms, he would not be missed by his grandchildren. As we grew older, we were told to call him and try to talk to him, an awkward obligation. As a young child, I saw that his participation in birthday celebrations was a UNICEF greeting card. I do not blame him for anything. He was just an old, aloof guy. He was a presence in the family in his last years mostly as a problem—how to manage his unhappiness and loneliness and find new caregivers for him.

To my father, the world is good. There must be some personal message in his father's suicide. My father's thinking ran something like, *Life is good, and I am in it. I am the most important relationship you have. Why do you want to get away from me? Why is being with me not enough to make your life worthwhile?* It absolutely does not compute with me that a middle-aged guy with his own kids in their teen years would take, what seems to me, the very rational suicide of his father personally. My father cannot see how pain, loneliness, and the knowledge that there is nothing but increasing pain and loneliness ahead—no new chapters in life, no new people, just assisted living, nursing home, hospice, and death—could make life a negative and death on one's own terms in one's own bed a reprieve. Even at age sixteen, though I had not experienced the loneliness and uselessness that comes with age, disability, and the death of those around you, I understood my grandfather.

I envied my grandfather in some respects. It took courage. The path of least resistance would have been to churn out another decade in loneliness to spare everyone else the burden and unpleasantness of suicide. That was not his style. He was the maverick of the family, leaving the family saloon and grocery business in Cleveland to live in rural California at the start of the twentieth century. He was a maverick in death. He had previously tried and failed to kill himself. He accepted the tut-tuts and admonitions of those around him not to do something so thoughtless. He was made to admit that he had acted foolishly and would not do it again. Ultimately, he acted for himself. That is how he spent his life, pursuing his own comfort without any passionate interest in those around him.

He really hurt nobody. He was lonely because nobody wanted him around on a regular basis. He was in a wheelchair, housebound, and most of his beautiful old California Spanish mystery maze of a house was inaccessible to him. Making new friends on his own was not a realistic possibility, and he would not have wanted to anyway. He was austere, well to do, but always choosing solitude and Arts and Crafts simplicity over a larger life. If those of us left behind are hurt, perhaps we are disappointed in ourselves. Had my grandfather been an active, wanted part of things—soccer games, decisions, the ups and downs of family life, sharing in movies and the other little pleasures along the way—he would not have lived in the isolation that made his life unpleasant. In truth, he did not want that, and those around him did not want that either.

I was very wrong about his death not hurting anyone in real, cutting terms. He hurt my father.

I hurt to see that my father was so wounded, that he believed there was a message to him in his father's death. I do not think my father could see it otherwise. He likes life. He cannot see the question as *Why should I live?* He can only see the question as *Why would I want to kill myself? Why would I ever want to leave my son?*

At the time of this trip, I was quite happy, but not as my father was. I was content. My meditation practice was strong. I felt like I was noticing everything, seeing how the millions of improbable bits of existence interconnected to construct our reality. I was open, seeing things clearly, difficult to perturb, disconnected from the push and pull, the slings and arrows of normal life. I had a foot in the infinite and could almost see entirely through the mountains and bison to the infinite forces creating and supporting them. My mind raced with endless interconnected facets of the world. My dad was happy to be in a pretty place and have a good steak, a content, constant, reliable person. Naturally wise.

Our conversation went through the topics of his father's suicide, what he might view as my possible suicide, his joys and disconnect with his father over his suicide, and happiness in general. You would think this would be some heavy soap-opera-like confrontation. It was not. We spoke freely and easily about ostensibly tough topics. I talked about my recent hospitalization, the revelations I felt I had through training my body and my new interest in mindfulness Buddhist practice, the comedy of having learned that I was not the first person to have my insights or look for a way to practice them. I talked about my path to happiness, believing at that time not just that I was well medicated but that I had cracked the code of the world. I told him I believed I had found some happiness and was on a path to sink more deeply into unshakable contentment. My story had a lot of work and twists and turns and drugs and learning and practice, but I think it will end with a slice of contentment.

My father found happiness more simply and easily. My father explained he has always been happy because he wanted to be happy. He said, "Happiness is a choice." He was happy because he decided to be happy. He could have chosen at many different points to be unhappy. His life had its disappointments, including his father's suicide. He chose not to be that guy. He decided he would be happy, and so he was. Amazing.

I find this provocative and think about it often. Is happiness a choice? There is immense wisdom packed into his outlook—choose to be happy. The phrase itself is immensely useful, and it now defines my father to me.

I imagine my father sitting with the Buddha. The Buddha sits under the bodhi tree, dramatic in his stillness, fist planted on the earth as he faces down every form of Mara. Every desire and temptation visit the Buddha—sex, wealth, status, fame—and somehow he has the balance and integration into all that is, a transcendence beyond expectation and desire, to resist everything. The Buddha's victory comes through a sort of passivity, but it is still a battle, and the Buddha is the hero winning a victory none of us could achieve. My father would sit in the same scene, content, enjoying the shade of the tree, enjoying the flow of gin into his veins, no battle, no heroism, just easy, effortless contentment. He is already at the transcendent finish line or happy enough and would not understand why Mr. Gautama was having such a hard time just sitting there on such a grand day. My father may not be fully enmeshed with the way of the universe, but he would appear to have the same ease sitting there, totally authentic to how he was created, no fighting or practice necessary.

Is happiness merely a choice? I cannot agree with my father entirely. Choosing to be happy is much of the story of becoming happy, but not the entire tale. For my father, it may be sufficient. He is extraordinary. For me it is helpful, essential, but incomplete.

Me: Happiness Is Not a Choice

I Did Not Choose My Brain

I have never been a happy person. I have always wanted to die. I would like to think that I have changed. I think I have seen contentment, but as Moses and MLK saw the mountain. I know it is there, but I know I will not get there. The truth is, I still struggle with suicide. Not wanting to die is conscious, daily work. The desire is always in my peripheral vision. The voice is always audible if I choose to listen. My life is usually a day-to-day affair, and sometimes I have justifiable fear that I will not make it through the night if I am left alone.

From my earliest memories, age three onward, I resented my parents terribly for having me. By what right did they bring me into the world, into a sentence of suffering? There was no problem until I was born. I would dream about and hope for death. The fantasies were very cartoonish, informed by TV programming for boys. Bad guy henchmen from the 1966 Batman TV show festooned with matching sweaters that said "Biff" and "Boff" would tiptoe into my room with a two-person timber saw and cut my head off, and then it would be over. They would run away with my head in a money sack, laughing with joy. (Why they wanted my head was never super clear.)

My basic coping mechanism was set truly from toddlerhood onward. As I lay in bed, trying to fall asleep, I would fantasize that someone would kill me, maybe even that night if I were lucky. I did not need to stress. I could relax. It was all temporary. I would be gone soon, and the misery would end with it. I could go back to however things were before I was born. I had no complaints prior to the year of my birth—1969. I could go back to 1968.

During the day, I was happy only when I was somebody else, usually Batman or Robin Hood. I was so attached to my costumes in nursery school that the teachers thought I had a problem. I had (and still have) a rich fantasy life. Even if part of my mind is consumed listening to and reacting to you in the shared world, much of my mind keeps the story of my alternate life going. Even when taking a test or doing something else that required present, complete concentration, I would mentally touch the fantasy—see the world of Snoopy or Robin Hood or Batman or *Star Wars*—many times per minute. In adulthood, it has generally been giving a peek to make sure all the colored jewel buttons on the bridge of the *Enterprise* are still blinking. Knowing another, happier world was there and would be there when I could return to it was a source of comfort.

My parents were overly doting, which, as problems go, does not a melodrama make. I grew up in an upper-middle-class home, a nice suburb about thirty-five miles east of downtown LA in a two-thousand-square-foot ranch house, and when I was in high school, my dad took out a loan and installed a Jacuzzi. There was no abuse, no hardship, no sad backstory. If one were looking to place blame, ninety percent of it would have to fall on the poison brew within my skull. It was there at the beginning and actually mellowed as time and external life difficulties grew. As a toddler I had an element of rage that quickly faded, less as a teen, and now none. There is no anger in this desire. It is a path to peace.

As I grew older, this unhappiness moved from infantile fantasy to more mature suicidal ideation. The only way I could get through life was to believe that sometime soon I would end it. Contemplation of an end and hope for an end moved into a desire for action. I never really tried to kill myself in a serious way as a kid. I would write a note, have a plan, pick a day. The day would come and go, and I would still be there, now filled with even more self-loathing because of my cowardice. I did this a number of times.

The hope of a near-term death has always been a balm that made life tolerable, even if I knew it was mostly fantasy. When in a poor frame of mind, it remains my go-to move and chief danger—writing down the minimum lethal doses of the drugs on hand on a Post-it note to carry with me, then getting the things assembled and accessible, and, ultimately, keeping a little bag of pills in my pocket I could pat whenever necessary.

As an older kid, nine through my teen years, I would punctuate my self-loathing for not ending things as planned with some petty act of self-harm. Stupid. Useless. The acts may leave me limping or nursing a small puncture wound for weeks, and that pain and inconvenience just served to remind me of my failures and unhappiness. That my parents and nobody else noticed just increased my isolation.

In law school, I received psychiatric treatment for the first time. The Harvard Law School clinic was made up, if memory serves, of one generalist and three psychiatrists. When you see HLS grads on TV, know that they are quite likely dysfunctional psych patients. I was overjoyed to have mental health care access for the first time. I had always known I needed it. My parents dragged me through or perhaps I directed them through rounds of exotic treatment as de-scribed above—I ate a sandwich with radioactive material injected in it, had stuff injected into my kidneys, tubes up my nose and down my throat and kept there for a day, hospitalizations, an unnecessary appendectomy, but all along I knew the problem was my mind. At each step, especially before they wheeled me off to have my belly cut open in the fourth grade, I wanted to shout, "This is not the problem. My brain is!" I never had the courage to do it. I knew physical sickness and demonstration of intelligence were what my mother valued in me. Intellectual and scholastic superiority supported my mother's standing publicly and drew her praise and pride at home. Physical illness won her attention and activity, gave her purpose and a vocation, an importance. I did not have the courage at age nine or even later to end the charade.

I assume my parents had too much of their ego invested in my general perfection to see or accept that my problems were psychiatric. I started taking antidepressants in law school, and I felt, I think, what it was like to be normalish. I was still a weirdo. I liked spending my time in BDSM nightclubs with Dominatrices. I still threw up and/or had diarrhea on the night before finals. My identity was so tight and fragile I could not manage the slightest failure. However, in moments, I could enjoy life too. With many things, I could take its ups and downs with appropriately sized emotions. I started doing plays, spending time with girls and indulging in kinky sex life in a serious way. This had always been a source of such shame; I never let myself live it. Sometimes the medications worked. Sometimes they did not.

When they did not, my depression matched my more mature stage of life. Things would get weird. I would live in the dark in my apartment half the time, sleeping and eating irregularly, which, in turn, moved depression into something more like psychosis than just being down. My identity was so strong, so rigid, and so totally dependent on getting good grades and being viewed as someone who got good grades that most of the time I could go about my life as a student doing well in school, having friends, and getting laid here and there. The fact that my life may have appeared normal from the outside increased my isolation and joylessness. I was not happy, except when I was, and this was a matter of chemistry and out of my control.

In hindsight, I see that extremely irregular periods of eating and sleeping, lack of sunshine, and a stressful vocation that was totally unsuited to my temperament and incompatible with what I liked were major factors, but none of those things felt like choices, like anything I could change. What, I was going to quit Stanford or Harvard just because I was miserable there, turn down title, prestige, and pay at an elite firm because I would rather work in the model shop than draft agreements for the studio? Tell everyone I am not smart and tough enough to make it in a man's world? The choices seem too wrong on the surface, and my unyielding, unipolar identity as an intellectual and achiever in things brainy would not permit it. I did not have the confidence required, and had I embarked on a different path, there simply would be nothing left of me. I would disappear.

A Lifelong Search for the Right Gun

My thoughts of suicide grew more dangerous in my dark periods. I came close while I was a summer associate in law school at the Newport Beach office of a white-shoe international law firm. For context, Newport Beach is a very nice place. It is where really rich guys go after they have become rich, often to be seen at right-wing fundraisers or driving around in Mercedes SLs with women younger than their daughters. I was thinking about skipping the first half of life and just start living as a really rich guy in Newport Beach immediately. Why not? My days consisted mostly of research projects and being taken out to dinner. Every Friday afternoon, the lawyers took over the rooftop of Hotel Laguna and got loaded on red wine right on the beach. (I am certain the firm's New York and London offices had no such traditions or a beach and sunset that could rival those of Laguna.) All of this, by most definitions, was winning. This was cashing in the chips of hard work for a dream life from age twenty-five forward.

Yet I was depressed and needed out desperately. I had a date, a spot where I was going to do it, a really well-written note (always an essential piece for me), and a method actually intended to work. There was no Rube Goldberg series of pills that if timed just so might carry me off with a smile on my face. No. This time, there was just a gun. I wanted to tie up every bit of work and every piece of my life, leave a clean desk, no email or voice mail unreturned, everything done, and nobody who could say I ducked out on anything or left them worse off. That is not easy to do, but I did it. I worked my inbox and life to a moment of total irresponsibility. I was in my beloved red Acura Legend feeling good that I was finally underway. I stopped at a gun shop in a lovely hell in the desert east of Orange County, where I would gaze into the horizon with an orchestral theme playing behind the moment and blow my brains out.

I had held and even fired handguns a few times before. Still, going through the guns was a startling experience. They felt unreasonably heavy. That was frightening. I did not realize how stiff the action on most guns is. I feared I could not bring myself to hold up the heavy gun and squeeze the trigger. It required a lot of will in the instant or some ability to distract myself from what I was doing long enough to get to that final Nike moment, to just do it. As I held the gun, I was already caught up in the cinematography in my mind, alone on the empty road with that gun in my hand. It was more tangible and vivid than a normal thought experiment. I was watching myself in at least two places at once. In the other place, there was a long instant of pulling the trigger, real effort. That interval and that effort were too much.

Back to my existence in the gun store, another gun, back to the desert, not right. Another gun, not right. I eventually told the store owner that I had a hand injury or some other thing that explained why I needed something easier to shoot without losing too much of my manly pride. I assumed he would move me from the giant magnum hand cannon the desert survivalists prefer to the ladies' purse guns. My fears of being emasculated were misplaced. He put a large revolver in my hand that had been modified, I would guess illegally, to have a hair trigger. I cocked the gun and barely pulled, not even a pull, just a meaningful tap. The hammer snapped down loudly. Touch. Snap. A loud mechanical snap, the force of the spring translated into a jarring noise with the very slightest volition and no physical effort. I was out in the desert and my brains were twelve feet from my body. I felt nauseous instantaneously.

I put the gun down and walked out. This all happened without thought.

It certainly is not my style to turn my back on someone and walk away without polite social pleasantries. I just knew when I touched the trigger and heard the snap that this was the gun, and if I left the store with it, I would be dead. I was shaken. I am not sure what I did after that, where I went, when I decided to go back home. I think I drove around the desert all day in a fugue state, trying to regain control of my breath. I scared the shit out of myself.

This was the closest I had come, a real plan executed up until the last step, a plan calculated to kill myself and partially experienced. I have played with suicide. Thought about it in circles so long I am bored with it and just tell my therapist to fill in the blanks. I have toyed with and a very few times done risky things, highly stupid things, but not things calculated to end my life for certain—enough pills and of a kind to risk death, but not guarantee it. At the scariest, my prior thoughts ran to *Let's do this, go to sleep, see what happens, nothing is for sure.* In fact, everything was calibrated not to be certainly fatal, just to risk death. If it were fatal for sure, I would not act. This time, in the desert, with that hacked gun, there was nothing risky. I would be dead. My head would be broken apart, and chunks of my brain would be oozing in the dust. This gun was an artillery piece, something out of a Clint Eastwood movie. There could be no grazing. It was guaranteed death even without a bullet. Definitive. Decisive. No mental games. No counting pills to roll the dice on a sleep becoming permanent. I walked up to the ledge and looked over. I held it. I heard what would be the last thing I would hear. I felt the last thing I would feel, and the trigger was so easy to pull. Touch. Snap. It took so, so, so little volition. No brooding. No long looks into the sunset. No starting to take pills and seeing how many I would down before unconsciousness. If I walked out of the shop with the gun, I would be dead. This episode was different.

Perhaps it was all just a more elaborate gesture, a bigger, more detailed show that I needed as my life descended into stress and what looked like decades of unhappiness ahead as a big firm lawyer.

However, failing to do the job, coming back alive was terrible. I returned to work. Everything mocked my existence. I should not have been there. Everything held the message that I would be miserable and was too cowardly to change my situation. The pattern for the coming decades was set. I did not mess with guns again, however.

After that unhappy youth, my life has been great in so many ways—enough money, titles, and prestige in every professional endeavor; learned and entertaining friends; nice houses; every car and geeky toy I have ever wanted; and most of all an amazing family, including two children who represent the pinnacle of creation, the purpose of the universe, and the end point of evolution. My life has been punctuated with wonderful experience as well, unremarkable but lovely trips to Italy, Israel, Hawaii, and beyond. I have enjoyed extraordinary adventures in learning, art, performance, and personal experience, beautiful and challenging, going down rabbit holes to find forms of pleasure, pain, and psyche and then learning about new rabbit holes to explore.

I have built up a war chest of reasons to live, yet I have engaged in risky behaviors in a game of Russian roulette with the world. I have overdosed and been hospitalized a number of times while having all of these things. I have hospitalized myself voluntarily because I could not trust myself through another long night, sitting alone with my own pessimism, self-hatred, and a voice demanding that I put the pills I had been carrying in my pocket as a security blanket into my mouth and do what, I thought, would be the right thing, so my family could go on and have a good life uninfected by my poison, so I could finally succeed, be the person I should be. I know how dangerous this is. These nights are as dangerous as a gun and a plan. It would just take a moment of pique or a what-the-fuck moment to pop the pills in my mouth. Then mad screaming and 911 as fear and regret would seize me, and a race between death and the hospital.

It is the unthinking moment, the moment when my mind is mostly elsewhere, that is so dangerous and unpredictable, not the heaviness of the metaphorical trigger. If the pills are in my hand and a big part of me just wants it to be over, hates myself for not taking action, one day, the pills will go into my mouth. That is how it went down with my one semiserious overdose. I was at home, miserable and distraught over an interrelated combination of financial and professional failures, radical emotional manipulation by a Dominatrix, and my typical insanity. I just started eating pills. Once I started, I realized I needed to keep going so I would die. I had no solid intention or plan. I had tripped into suicide. I was terrified, but I had to go forward. It became clear that I could not stay awake to get enough of the drug in me. I was very familiar with what doses caused what effect. I would wake up with severe liver damage, debilitated, and this was never a goal. I called out for help. Then it was a nurse slapping me and yelling at me, charcoal, you have seen it all on TV.

I had planned over-the-top dramatic deaths . . . once at Point Loma in San Diego, a beautiful spot overlooking the ocean. I took it all in, a final run on the cliffs, but the place I wanted to be had other people there. I ran around looking for a nice spot, and everywhere there were people. It is so stupid, but I did not want my final moments to be listening to drunk teenagers. That defeated the high drama of the death-at-sunset Point Loma plan. (Maybe in the winter I could put something together with my hands, releasing a dove as I expire à la *Blade Runner*.) I got frustrated and went home. I know none of this makes sense. It surely means that I had no settled, determined desire to end my life. I cannot explain why I have been caught in cycles of effete, juvenile near disasters, hospitalizations, and overdoses rather than ordinary life or funerals. All so stupid.

Mental Illness Is Not a Choice

I do not think I chose any of this. I am insane. My brain has aberrant neurochemical properties that do this. I am unhappy. Living is hard for me. In my natural state, a voice is always telling me to kill myself. This is not typical, and it is not choice. I know because when I take a pill that changes the brain chemistry, I am a different person, happy, sometimes ecstatic. I have walked through the world whistling and smiling until my face muscles fatigued because I took the right pill or too much of the right pill. I have walked through the world in darkness with the wrong pills in my pocket. I have strode along singing a tune, eager to give a hail-fellow-well-met to anyone I encounter. I have stewed in the darkness, hoping we humans somehow destroy ourselves so the dogs take over. This is chemistry. Not choice.

There are environmental and behavioral factors that create or exacerbate the brain's unhappy orientation. For me, sleep and food deprivation are the things that ramp up the misery of being alive. However, it is a preexisting problem that makes me think not eating for two days is a good idea. There is a spiral of neural dysfunction through behavior and back to an even worse-off brain.

I have been stable on a cocktail of drugs for a number of years with only tinkering of dosages here and there, maybe throwing in a new pill now and then, tweaks, not changes. I have been generally sane for a long time. This is neurochemistry. I would like to think that the way I have lived and learned is responsible. It is not. I could not have started down the path of observing, acting, and understanding without the stability and baseline happiness brought by the chemicals.

If you have gone into a hospital because you cannot keep from physically attacking yourself in delusions that such an action is necessary or a good idea, or if you are simply so miserable existing and you want the pain to end so much that you're given a pill and skip out of the hospital singing show tunes, mystified about who it was that entered the hospital, you know it is chemistry, not choice. We do not choose to have off-kilter serotonin or dopamine processes any more than a diabetic chooses not to make insulin.

It is hard for others to see and accept mental illness in someone around them. I have Parkinson's disease. My shortage of important neurotransmitters usually translates into tremors, slowness, and other movement symptoms. Nobody would say this was my choice. It is no different with mood disorders, psychosis, and a host of other things. My lack of dopamine in a different context within the brain would change other processes, like mood and more social behaviors. It is not choice. The manifestations are just behaviors that seem to have a large element of choice to a brain functioning in the typical way. Nobody chooses to have a hand tremor. Not many people have a tremor. The tremor has the flavor of an illness. Everyone experiences bad moods and acts unwisely. This has the feel of life in general and things directed by free will.

It is also difficult to see mental illness in oneself, even when confronted with objectively true, irrefutable evidence. We cling to a sense of self that is essentially the operation of these processes—our moods, our emotions, our outlook, how we act in different situations. Most people would say that is personality itself. To accept mental illness is to accept that we are not who we think we are or that we are not there at all, just a chemical soup inside a skull.

Acknowledging our physical existence is a threat. We want to see ourselves as embodied angels, mini gods in command of a machine. The machine, the body, may be injured and will quit working, but we are not that machine. We are some kind of invisible homunculus controlling the machine. To move forward, you have to let go of this idea of self. It is too false and unstable to be useful. To see mental illness, you need to let go of this aggrandizing sense of self.

Our brains make the world and who we are. Our brains construct our reality. Even the most basic things like shape, size, and color are constructs. For some people the brain constructs a livable home. For others it does not. It is not choice.

To this extent, my father's view that happiness is a choice is demonstrably false. However, this is not the full story, and to someone with a brain that lets them function with a normal range of emotions, mental illness is not part of the story at all. From where my father sits, a super affable, well-adjusted guy who could probably sit with a smile on his face during a nuclear apocalypse, this is true. Happiness is a choice. My father was not bad, stupid, or even wrong. That was his reality. If one has a typically functioning brain, in fact, my father's view holds a great deal of wisdom. He was right for himself. He could more or less will himself to be happy. Amazing.

Perhaps my father and I represent extremes. My father was someone so naturally affable and at ease with himself and the world that contentment was his natural state. He had to look away to be unhappy. Being depressed was work, so being happy was an easy choice. He just had to go on about his business. That is a doable, simple decision, and voilà, happiness returns effortlessly. I have been naturally unhappy. Staying aboveground has been a struggle. I am forever fighting my natural internal state and interpretation of the world. Survival is work. Doing what I need to do to be a father, husband, and friend is work. Happiness is possible and achievable, but it is a life's work, daily effort, hourly effort. I cannot choose to be happy and be happy. If Jeannie from *I Dream of Jeannie*, Q from *Star Trek*, and Uncle Martin from *My Favorite Martian* all blinked, snapped their fingers, and pointed at the same time, they could not teleport me to happiness. I cannot choose to be happy or made happy absent the right modifications to my brain.

However, this is not the story: there is no choice. My father is normal and can be happy at will. I am insane and can never be happy. My story emphatically does not end there. In the last ten years, I started to run and grew healthy, in part, to continue the enjoyment of my artistic and erotic interests. The much larger motivation was the understanding acquired when grounded in settled moments of what would actually happen to my young children if I were to disappear. This was not really about me anymore. My existence was necessary for the happiness of my children. I had to live. So I became a student of living, which includes observation and understanding of when psychiatric intervention is useful, but also what can be done by the day, hour, and moment to continue life. That path has pushed my life out far longer than I would have thought possible. My new vocation as a student of being has also given me glimpses of serenity, real happiness, deep contentment, and tiny tastes of transcendence. That keeps me going.

I have learned that while happiness is not there for the taking, I can do things to engender happiness—exercise, meditate, modify my thinking, observe the world, and learn, among other things. I can choose to do these things. So to be happy, I must make a choice to pursue happiness. In fact, my path requires greater conviction and discipline; the choice must be stronger precisely because it runs against the grain of biology and personality.

Is happiness a choice? Probably not for most people. I do not think there are a lot of David Grossmans out there who can choose to be happy and be happy without any intermediate steps. However, happiness for everyone requires choice. However easy or hard the decision and the work that follows, with a typically functioning brain or an aberrant one, comfortable circumstance or harsh, to be happy, one must choose to be happy and take steps to engender happiness.

Happiness requires a choice—to pursue happiness.

CHAPTER 15

How to Choose Happiness

You cannot simply choose to be happy. You can, however, think and act in ways that are likely to lead to happiness. You can change yourself and the circumstances around you in positive ways, increasing your chances of happiness. You can also change your thinking. Adopt an outlook that frames the facts of your world to maximize happiness. Both of these moves—thinking and doing—to make one happy engender positive, virtuous cycles, where the pursuit of pain produces swirling cycles of misery all the way down the drain.

You Have Choice

Happiness is not a choice per se, but achieving happiness requires wise choices. Almost every thought presents an opportunity to choose happiness or to walk away from happiness. This entire treatise on life and the universe and everything can be viewed as an instruction manual on how to figure out what will make one happy, choose to do that thing, do it, repeat cycle. Goals, the path to them, and the trip itself are just a means of finding happiness.

For most animals and some people, there is not much room for choice. Every moment is a struggle for survival. There is not time for contemplation, and most choices are Hobson's choices at best. Spend twenty hours per day looking for food and shelter or you will die hungry and cold. If you have the leisure time and interest to read this, this is not you. Your circumstances are not that constraining.

Does choice exist? We might as well live as if it does. I cannot make an argument for actual free will. I see no logical basis for believing that we really can choose A or B. However, I do not see how this likely lack of free will changes our *feeling* of free will or how we should act in any circumstance. You have a mind to observe your situation and choices to make in response to that world in light of whatever you are trying to achieve. You could say that choice and what you choose to do represent the free will of the angel who lives inside you. You could point to a course of events whose history was written at the big bang. Either way, it does not matter in the life of the individual. The subjective experience is the same.

How you think about things has a great deal to do with whether those things engender joy, fear, or any other emotional reaction. You can frame your reality with thoughts that encourage happiness. You can choose to think about the world and about what you are doing in ways that bring happiness.

Reframe the Situation in Your Mind

Willie Shakes, through dazed, confused, and suicidal Hamlet, wrestles with and nails all the big existential questions:

> HAMLET
> Denmark's a prison.
>
> ROSENCRANTZ
> Then is the world one.
>
> HAMLET
> A goodly one; in which there are many confines,
> wards and dungeons, Denmark being one o' the worst.

ROSENCRANTZ
We think not so, my lord.

HAMLET
Why, then, 'tis none to you; for there is nothing
either good or bad, but thinking makes it so: to me
it is a prison.

ROSENCRANTZ
Why then, your ambition makes it one; 'tis too
narrow for your mind.

HAMLET
O God, I could be bounded in a nut shell and count
myself a king of infinite space, were it not that I
have bad dreams.

Nothing is either good or bad, but thinking makes it so.

Whether something is a source of happiness or pain is largely a matter of thinking and expectations, things within one's own control. This is probably the most practical and powerful advice I have to offer: **You can control the way you think about something, and how you think about something shapes the way you feel.** I view this as the crux of cognitive behavioral therapy. It is astonishing how with a tiny twist of thought, reframing the situation, one's emotions change. You cannot control whether someone almost kills you on the freeway. You can control whether you feel rage or gratitude in the situation by choosing how you think about the incident. You can control whether to continue on your drive enjoying the mellow tunes of AM radio or to carry anger with you through everything you do, even trying to sleep.

This is so easy and so powerful. How you frame the situation in your mind determines what you feel—whether pleasure or pain. Feeling, therefore, changes instantly with thought. You can choose to reframe the situation in your mind in a way that induces happiness—a choice to be happy or something very close to it.

I have found several ways to reframe situations extremely effective, some being more suitable than others in a particular circumstance. I think of these as moves, tricks, jukes in the mind, ways to give anger and melancholy a head fake and sprint toward happiness, leaving everything negative behind.

Something crappy or triggering happens. Someone is terrible to you and others. The Fates scream down a situation bound to thwart your plans and cause pain. There are several ways you can modify your thinking to reframe the situation so experience tilts toward happiness.

Focus on the Objective

In any situation, when the fury starts to rise, you can choose to ask yourself, "Does this in any way impede what I am doing?"

A driver cuts you off, violating all laws and etiquette, almost killing you. You and the driver behind skid to a violent stop on the freeway to avoid collision. To make it extra spicy, I'll throw in that he believed you were Hispanic, flipped you off, and screamed, "Go back to Mexico," as he caused this possibly fatal situation, leaving the MAGA, NRA, and Blue Lives Matter stickers on his truck as the last things you may see in this life.

You live and are back on your way in moments.

Does this turn of events impact you and what you are doing? No.

Does it keep you from reaching your big goal pinned on the calendar months from now? No.

Does it impede your ability to do whatever you need to do that day to reach that goal? No.

Does it keep you—you personally without looking at things at a social level—from doing anything you intended to accomplish that day, that hour? No.

Even if driving somewhere is your immediate objective, this near-death experience and collision with an antisocial asshole who hates you without reason has no impact. It is a nullity, irrelevant to everything you are doing.

Can you choose not to be angry? Not directly unless beatification may be in your future. You can, however, even if angry, choose to ask yourself whether the situation impacts your goals and activity and go through an analysis that leads to an answer. If the answer is no, this incident and jerk have no impact, and the otherwise infuriating experience that might hang with you for days becomes an irrelevancy. Its irrelevancy saps its power to control you. Your focus moves away from it and stays on what you should be doing. This guy's actions, dangerous, hate-filled, and antisocial as they are, will not get to you. None of it matters. This will leave you as content as you were before. You may even be happy, grateful to be alive. You will be vastly happier than you would be if you made this guy, people like him, how their ignorance and hate kills, an intimate companion nestled in your head, an ongoing source of anger.

You can choose to ask the questions and think through to an answer in less than five seconds and buy your emotional freedom for days.

Let Go of What Is Out of Your Control

Even if some circumstance is in your way, you can ask yourself if there is anything you can do about it. It could be something small (traffic on the 405 that could make you late) or something big (you have cancer and need to get your affairs in order, as the euphemism goes). This move always has great power.

You know that it is highly stupid to get angry or even have feelings about things out of your control. Some people get angry at the weather. If you ask yourself whether there is anything you can do (about the weather, traffic, or even cancer) that you are not doing and the answer is *No, I cannot do anything more to do what I need to do,* you have removed yourself from the situation. You are acknowledging that you would be effectively getting angry at the weather (God? The laws that govern barometric pressure?). Your anger has no purpose and is foolish. If you fall, should you get angry about gravity, get really pissed that you are not in another universe where masses repel each other?

Equanimity flows from an acknowledgment that what is happening is totally out of our hands. You cannot always choose not to feel angry when you find yourself in traffic, but you *can* choose to ask yourself if there is even an ounce of sanity in your reaction. If there is not, if the traffic is out of your control, contentment flows from your answer. If you accept that traffic is out of your control, your pointless urge for it to change will dissipate. Banging on the steering wheel will seem silly.

You can move your mind to more practical and positive matters. You will be happier. Choose to ask the right questions, to put your mind in the proper place with the answers.

With practice, this process can be instantaneous, faster than words. With practice, it is a nonverbal general outlook, and with more practice, that outlook can become your default way of looking at things. You will not need to ask yourself the question, because the traffic just will not make you angry. You need not have a reaction at all if you deeply internalize what is out of your control.

Release Things in the Past

For me, accepting past mistakes is a major problem. I still spend way too much time keeping myself from happiness because of something I said in high school or professional decisions I made that turned out poorly (e.g., I was asked to interview at Pixar very early in the company's history, and I turned it down). I stew over the past and dig into self-loathing, forgetting the interesting, exciting, successful life I have had because I was embarrassed in the past. I rue things that happened in the eighth grade, and I am fifty-three.

What has happened is out of your control. That is true. It is in the same bucket as the weather. Sure, it was your error, but time moves in only one direction for you. You can only change what you do in this moment and the next one. Yet, I torture myself.

The first mental move does not work for me. The past mistake does not feel and may not be irrelevant. The mistake has an impact on how I view myself today, and when it comes to some specific mistakes, the mistake changed my life course. I have made so many. I am fortunate, but peers of mine became billionaires doing basically the same thing as I did, but picking the right job where I picked the wrong one (I will die waiting for my Q4 1999 IPO payoff when it seemed that money was raining down on everyone). Sometimes I torment myself for not taking a path more similar to my peers, one that I wanted to pursue at one time but rejected, and then they ended up in the Senate or on the federal bench. They made smarter moves. The bizarre thing is I would not trade lives with any of them given the choice. It is all a pointless means of self-torment. I play with my kids, hang out at Disneyland, go to vampire balls and other silly events, play how I want to play without care over my image or standing, and write.

I do tell myself that these memories I regurgitate to torment myself are just that, evanescent chemical chains imprinted by something that is out of my control. It helps, but I still struggle a great deal here. If I were to identify one central character flaw, it is that my default position is hatred of myself. It is difficult to distract myself from that core identification, thoughts worn into grooves in my brain like the trenches in Roman roads carved by hundreds of thousands of carts over thousands of years. It is hard to get the wheel out of the trench.

All I can say on this point is don't do it. Don't dig the comfortable trench of self-loathing. Don't take yourself that seriously. There is nothing to lament if things turn out okay, and even if you have made serious, damaging mistakes, there is truly nothing to do but learn and move on. Time is a one-way ticket on a one-way metaphorical train. You can pull the cord, scream at the conductor, or jump off the train, but the train cannot go backward to a stop you missed.

Move to Another Objective

Sometimes you really will hit a hard roadblock. You will not be able to do what you want to do in the short term (e.g., go to the concert you have been waiting to see for ten years because there were no tickets available or it was canceled). You may lose your long-range goal or general life direction. You are training for the Rome Marathon, and back problems and surgery are keeping you from it, and longer term, your body does not permit you to run again. (That sounds familiar.) There is only one solution in the face of hopes hitting a real wall. In the case of the concert, you will need to change your weekend plans. In the bigger picture, you will need to change what goal you are working toward and more generally what activity composes your life. It happens.

When you hit a wall, you must switch to a new objective. You can even frame the roadblock and need to change as an opportunity. You cannot go to the show? Accept it. That's real fact. But neato, I can go out with my pal. I finally have the window to make that happen. You cannot make it to the marathon or maybe run again? Pain, but this opens up the time to write and creates new motivation to live out your ambition to write.

Writing this, it does sound Pollyannaish: "It ain't so bad; we could use these sheets as curtains and the barn as the theater; we will put on the show anyway. Isn't it grand that I have lost the ability to do the only thing I find rewarding and fun?" Still, give the tactic a go. It has been a useful and effective mental move.

You cannot do x. Losing x is not altogether bad, because now you get to do y. Working on y, x goes from disappointment to irrelevancy or even opportunity. If one door closes, walk through another one. You may need to create the new door, but stagnation and disappointment is the only other option.

All these ways to reframe the situation dance around the same core dynamics. You can choose how you think about your circumstances, and different thoughts lead to different emotional reactions.

Do Not Add Villains to Your Story

There are facts, and then there are interpretations of facts. It is easy to confuse the two. Often, the facts themselves are neutral, but we choose to make them problematic by ascribing bad motives to actors, assuming bad outcomes from the facts, and otherwise casting the pall of a darkness within our own personality on the world. There is a Buddhist story I bring to mind all the time and find very helpful in turning anger into contentment or even compassion.

A man is piloting his boat down a river. An irresponsible boatman crashes into him. The man is irate. He screams at the offending boatman. He carries his anger with him the rest of the day. The offending boatman moved on happily, forgetting the incident, but the hero of the parable gives up his happiness and remains angry for hours, his mind running off on tangents of how the kids are not properly trained these days, the disrespect the other boatman showed him, and on and on. He is unhappy. If a stray log in the river were to bump into our boatman in exactly the same manner as the boat piloted by our irresponsible, drunk, negligent, mean fool, the boatman would not be angry at the log. His day continues unaffected. Change boats and pilots to cars and drivers and you have the exact story of freeway rage and the best solution for it.

The negative emotion stems from ascribing motives and personality to the problem. Our boatman is angry not because his boat was knocked but because he has made the other boatman a hostile villain. If he chose not to ascribe any motive or characteristics to the other boatman, he has nobody over whom to fume. There is no bad guy out to get him. There is just a log with a guy sitting on top of it.

If you cannot accept that there was no human motive behind something that harms you, you can choose to hypothesize motives that do not make you angry. Someone cuts you off speeding; maybe they are racing their pregnant wife to the hospital. Even if someone is just being a jerk, you do not know their story. They could be overtaxed by caring for a loved one at home. They could be mean because they are mentally ill. You do not know what is going on in the body, mind, and life of this other person, so choose to tell a story about him that does not make you angry.

Even if we assume the guy is just a jerk, getting angry harms only you. He could be a factor in your life keeping you awake as a fantasy in your head. To him, you were another of thousands of cars on the freeway he saw that day, unremarkable, irrelevant. You are not in any kind of conversation with this person. There is zero reason to look at things in a way that keeps an unpleasant person in your life. You are not in his head. You are the only combatant in this unnecessary and imaginary fight. Choose an interpretation that lets the jerk leave your life as quickly as he entered. You are the only one harmed.

Do not ascribe negative motives or, for that matter, *any* motives to those around you.

It Is Not Misfortune. It Is the World.

There is a wonderful Buddhist parable that I deploy as a coping mechanism for problems great and small. A man has a glass bauble that he loves. It is beautiful. He carries it with him everywhere he goes, and his love for it never wanes. He is even known as the man with the lovely glass orb. The prized bit of glass eventually rolls off a table and breaks irreparably. Those around the man gasp, expecting rage or sorrow for the destruction of something so important to him. When asked why he was not upset, he remarked that the glass was already broken when he got it.

When things seem bad, even bad on a cosmic scale—you have cancer and will die—you can choose to look at your situation in the context of the cosmic reality. You will die. That is the nature of being a human. The glass orb of your life was broken upon conception. Your death and most likely your sickness leading to death were effectively burned into the script the day you came to be. You are human. You are not immune.

Very bad things happen to people, the good people and the bad people alike. If what seems like ill fortune befalls you, it really is not bad luck. The universe was not unfair to you. These bad things do happen. That is the nature of the world. It happened to you. You are not immune. Here, I imagine my grandma Nettie pushing my arm and saying, "What? You think the sun shines out of your ass? Too good to have anything bad happen? Didn't anyone teach you? You got shit for brains or something?"

We should all keep this concept handy. Bad things will happen. It is a certainty. It is the nature of the world. It is the nature of being human. I find this approach very helpful in bits of bad luck big and small—the air-conditioning breaking on the hottest week of the year, needing to buy a new one for $11,700, and the pain throughout the week of trying to get the company to deliver and install it as my family melts.

It is less poetic, but in the place of the glass orb, you can drop in an air-conditioning compressor, a leaky roof, the cracked engine of a beloved car, or anything else.

The air-conditioning compressor was already broken when it was installed. What did you expect? You thought you could live in a desert for the rest of your life and you would not have to replace it? Only a tragic early death would prevent living through the compressor replacement. From Nettie, "What's wrong with you? *Meshuggener!* You think Moses blessed your compressor on Sinai, your thirty-year-old compressor was never going to break with temps over 105 for a week? Shit for brains." (She liked saying "shit for brains.")

One notable Buddhist teacher has a good move. He tells himself in such situations that most would consider misfortune, "This is being human. I am not immune." These are things that happen, and they can happen to you.

We live in a state of constant denial. It is bizarre that we have a difficult time internalizing the most basic inevitability of life—death and quite likely sickness and pain along the way.[23] People get cancer and get into terrible car crashes. We see that in the news all the time. It happens to other people all around us and their families. People around us die. For privileged Westerners, we may see it a few times in a lifetime with our own family and friends, wonder why it happened, and then forget that it happened. We generally do not believe these things—pain, sickness, death, or injury—will happen to us. Somehow, on some level, we get through each day with a sub silentio understanding that pain, sickness, and death are for other people, not us. None of us is immune. Bad things all the way up to a prolonged painful death or an untimely early death happen to people. You should not be surprised or angry if something bad happens not just to people in the news, but to you as well.

---

23. I am sure it is a very different story for the less fortunate for whom disease and death are a present part of daily life. The willful ignorance or blindness to unpleasant aspects of life applies to people secure enough in life to find the greatest stressors in a climate-controlled office and whose entire involvement with death is calling an undertaker a few times to pick up a body. Seeing pain and suffering must change perspective. This is the starting point in the ethical progress of the Buddha: the prince with the charmed life begins his quest for understanding upon seeing age, decay, and death for the first time. In Thailand, Buddhist monks enjoy a legal privilege to watch autopsies. Seeing bodies opened and the chunks inside removed and plated must be a powerful reminder that one's own body is full of chunks that can and will be removed and plated. It would be an instructive regular exercise for everyone. American culture would consider the exercise obscene, disrespectful to the dead, the desire to watch a sign of insanity, and the whole notion generally immoral. In addition to our privileged removal from the harsh truths of nature, we face a cultural edifice constructed to conceal the most certain truths of nature and make observing them deviant or criminal.

This is being human—I am not immune. Neither are you.

The Strange Reactions to My Diagnosis

My experience being diagnosed with Parkinson's has dropped me into this denial of sickness in a new way, now from the inside. I have told my wife, kids, three friends, and my psychiatrist. I figured it would get weirder and more difficult to bring up as time went on. This is what I have. This is why my hand shakes, I cannot write, and so on. Down the road you will see other symptoms manifest. Here is what they likely are. Done. No secrets. Done. All info out while it is easy to get out. Nothing more to discuss. The reaction tended to be "Oh my God. How are you doing? How can I help? Are you okay?" It seems so strange because I am not at all perturbed.

I have carried much tougher diagnoses before this. I should make it into and maybe through my seventies, maybe, with an okay life. People are told they have brain cancer and three months to live all the time. When I take my little one to see their doctor at Children's Hospital LA, so many of the children and families I see would sacrifice anything to be in my shoes. Perfect tiny children get sick and die, tormented with treatments they could not understand. Parents tie balloons to the beds of their insensible children, pretending that somehow it is okay, a normal family, a happy birthday celebration. I sneak off into the men's room and cry.

But I am not saying feel good because some other sucker has it worse. My thought process and feeling for me are simply *This happens. People get sick and die. We are all decaying.* This is how it is happening to me, at least in part. I have no cause for complaint. (To whom would I be complaining? Is there a single parent at Children's Hospital who would find my story interesting? My story is not interesting.) I feel fortunate. There is actually a shade of happiness in the diagnosis. It is not so bad. Ideally, I would be able to feel this way when I am told my death is imminent. I am working toward that. I think I am in a good place, but I will not know how I fare until tested. I am merely human. I am not immune.

Reframe Everything with a Positive Outlook

You can approach any situation with a positive outlook. As Hamlet tells us rightly, in most things, it is merely your thinking that makes something good or bad, so choose to consider things good. Even arduous tasks can be mentally framed to make them fun. For some, it is even possible to turn pain into something desirable. Work and play, pleasure, and some forms of pain are labels we get to put on things ourselves.

Mary Poppins put it more lyrically, to paraphrase:

> In every job you have to do
> There is something fun
> You find the fun and the job's a lark.

This does not require years of training; just choose to look at things, even things that are more easily characterized as bad, positively. Attitude. Outlook. These have a big impact. Forcing a smile has a big impact on mood. The forced smile translates into an easy smile, which modifies mood and how we process the facts of a situation. Medical research has demonstrated the positive impact the act of smiling has on mood as a matter of brain chemistry.

Many times per day we have a choice so subtle we usually do not even recognize that we are making a decision. If it feels like you can just choose to be happy, it is because you are going into something with a positive attitude, and that attitude is the feeling of happiness for you. It is not quite choosing to be happy directly, but extremely close. In fact, you are *choosing* to look at things positively, and adopting that outlook reframes the situation to highlight the positive and overlook the negative. This seems like a distinction without a difference, and I think that is true for a person functioning in the typical way. I am in a good mood. The world is good. For someone with a mood disorder, even if it were possible to have a positive outlook, which itself takes work, coming out on the other end feeling happy without any other intervention is unlikely.

For a good natured, well-balanced person like my father, a positive outlook is effectively choosing to be happy. To them, there is no question or confusion about wanting happiness. Of course, they want it. Any sort of rut, such as a mind mired in depression or anger, is alien. They have little difficulty in imposing a positive point of view. They can let themselves be angry or sad, and after a few hours or days, they smack the dust off their hands and say, "That's enough of that. I'm going to stop this negative stuff. I'm moving on now." The leap from outlook to mood is nonexistent. Inclined to hold on to a positive outlook, they do not have to do any mental work to impose that outlook on facts and have the resulting happiness outweigh the building pressure of a negative move. They have been dealt a bad hand, and they decide to smile and keep singing "Walking on Sunshine."

There was a lovely woman who managed the word processing center of my first law firm during the graveyard shift. I would be suffering, stressed, exhausted, thinking Job did not know anything about misfortune. At 3:00 a.m., there could be an asshole attorney feeling that their career and sanity hung in the balance, leaning over her, demanding that she go faster, being overly critical and intolerant of predictable mistakes, that she assign more people to their job. Sometimes there would be a motorcycle messenger dressed like an anime ninja in a multicolored leather jumpsuit standing by, looking at his watch, saying, "I can no longer guarantee that your document makes it to the LAX post office on time and be stamped before midnight." The stress on attorneys is immense, and these particular attorneys, while not abusive, were hardly their best selves.[24] She was the least senior person in the conversation, but she had an equanimity, always a smile, imperturbable. A smile. Always a huge smile. She had a sign up in her cubicle: "Too Blessed to Be Stressed." What a great way to be. The way she kept her poise, her calm, and her smile when all around her were melting down and their stress ended up falling on her as

---

24. Since I liked to loiter in the word processing center, I often overheard the frank conversation among the ladies (yes, I think they were still all women, and I think they were still mostly African American too—a different world). After an encounter with a decomposing attorney, the chatter would run to "I would not be an attorney for any amount of money," "Life is too short to be that guy," and so on. This is in the context of gargantuan pay disparities, someone making well over one million dollars to someone making well under one hundred thousand dollars. I envied them.

basically a lower-ranked person is an example I keep with me. It had the knock-on effects of protecting her people from the difficult situation, letting them just do their jobs unimpeded, and lowering the temperature for everyone. Perhaps I remember her so well because she brought me some sense of confidence and peace in difficult times, at 4:00 a.m., when it seemed my career, education, and identity were crashing. I looked forward to going into the windowless room packed with people typing away because I would get to talk to her and see her smile that pushed back against the slings and arrows of life. Her warm smile that could light a football stadium. I do not remember entirely what she looked like, but I remember the "Too Blessed to Be Stressed" sign and her smile.

Having this general desire to see things positively and to be happy may be a necessary precursor to all of the foregoing tactics. Maybe you will not get to the level of which trick works the best until you have the desire to smile, to be happy. Logically, that seems correct, but it does not match my subjective experience. I go to the tactics because my outlook is negative and things seem hopeless. My outlook is not positive, but I retain a portion of my mind not shoved about by the situation and my negative interpretation of it. I retain some objectivity. It is the voice out of nowhere in a marathon that tells me to stop, remove myself mentally from the moment, and try to reconceptualize the situation. This changes my outlook. For me, training my mind to remove my personality from the situation and arrive at an objective understanding allows me to put my situation together in my mind in a way to engender happiness.

For me, there is work at every step: find an objective understanding, choose to pursue happiness, deploy various tactics to engender happiness, repeat cycle. At my father's funeral, I spoke about his ability to choose to be happy and to simply be happy, instantly, without other steps or intermediate work. I spoke about how alien we were to each other. I spoke about how I wanted to be him and still do. I am not him, but I believe I can get to the same place. With effort, I can choose to pursue happiness. I can then do the work that engenders happiness. I can continue to work until I find it.

There is a choice to pursue happiness. There is also work to get there.

CHAPTER 16

Pursuing Happiness Is Itself a Life Discipline

To move forward toward happiness, one must decide to pursue happiness. This, like so much else here, seems too obvious to state, yet it is the fundamental failure point for many. It has been for me.

I have wasted years of life because I did not choose to be happy. If you had asked me if I wanted to be happy, I would have said of course. I am not the hairshirt, suffer-for-the-sake-of-heaven sort. At the same time, I was not shaping my life to pursue happiness, and pursuing happiness was not present as a goal in day-to-day decision-making.

Fight the Temptation to Return to Negative Mental States

There is a temptation to fall back to conflict and anger as the way we understand our situation and how we motivate ourselves to act. Why do we look to anger to move us forward? It is a sign of general human derangement and cultural insanity that this is the default outlook for many people, I would guess most people in America. So many people love feeling aggrieved so much their wealth and privilege are invisible, or if visible, they are aggrieved because if there were any justice, they would have more. There are a lot of gloomy Camerons. Lots of angry Trump people collecting their social security checks, kept comfy and alive with Medicare, yet absolutely infuriated at racial and ethnic minorities paying the taxes that support them. Why? Why would you be wealthy, retired, have limited years left, and want to be angry so badly you create a fantasy world where you and your world are victims. Why would you fabricate a world you believe to be unfair that leaves you unjustly wounded and impotent? Racism is never going away so long as people want to feel aggrieved, and there is a category of people separated by skin color or other identifying traits on whom to blame their untethered anger.

Positive political and policy views rooted in reality often still lean on anger—anger at the unfair biases of the racists, income inequality, poverty, disease, and danger in so much of the world, and a laundry list of other injustices that should be fixed. These are real and horrible wrongs, but why do we go to anger? Why do we imagine our work for justice as a "war on poverty," "war on cancer," always a war? Why is feeding a continuing unhappiness the default motivation for acting? Is acting to achieve a positive end because it is a positive end more difficult than leaning on burning anger to reach a positive end? It is odd, considering that the wisdom literature throughout the millennia, many of the nonviolent heroes we venerate, and the personal experience of so many people demonstrate the self-destructive nature of anger and negative emotions. They can be powerful motivators, but they come at a high cost.

I am still trying to sort out my recent, very personal running experience where I resorted to anger and negative emotion. I am left with mixed thoughts. I achieved what I wanted to achieve, and what I wanted to achieve was a lot. Anger took me across many finish lines I should not have been crossing. Doing so felt very good. However, I may have broken myself, perhaps beyond complete repair. I felt good throughout because I constructed a fantasy world chock full of powerful cultural memes that resonate with me, and in that fantasy world I had constructed and in which I chose to live, I triumphed. The fantasy has ended, and I am left with an unhappy reality.

I knew better. My meditation practice was pretty good by my standards. I believed I had attained some wisdom, a clear view of what was happening and an equanimity in navigating my circumstances. I am not writing anything I did not understand at the time. I lost all of it so quickly, intentionally, with knowledge of what I was doing. I knew I was acting unwisely, contrary to everything I believed I had figured out as matters of knowledge and skills of life practice. I did it anyway because it felt so good. It worked for a time too.

I was faced with circumstances I did not like. Things were not going well for me and seemed to be declining at a pace faster than I had assumed. It felt like I was losing everything. I had to skip a marathon. I was seeing double and getting dizzy when I ran. At my last race, I ran with one eye shut much of the time and hunched over to see curbs and bumps in the road. There were bigger changes too. My life, my personality, my mind, everything seemed to be changing for the worse. I was slowing down, physically and cognitively. There were rounds of doctors and tests. All of this I have told you before. My psychiatrists were attacking things with their own arsenal of drugs. There were no conclusive tests of anything. Each expert I saw doled out a diagnosis. My life seemed over. Perhaps the inherent cruelty of the universe wanted to make sure I withered for years as a dolt because I had lived as an intellectual looking for a quick way out. I was unhappy. My fortress of books and ramparts of sheepskin mocked me.

The rapid decline ended as suddenly as it began. With the help of high doses of steroids, I awoke. I was me again. It was like waking up from a bizarre dream where I had inhabited someone else's reality. I was awake, but I did not know how long the day would last. It seemed to be a gift. I decided I was going to see my dear friends immediately while I could move and talk lucidly. Then, after saying hellos and potential goodbyes, I was going to run, run, and run as long as my body would permit. I wanted to use up my body on a course before I lost it to some vague failure of cells doing this or that. At age forty-nine, in what I feared would be a small window of health, I ran six races, including my fourth marathon, in six months. (I also completed two running challenges—Conquer LA and the Beach Cities Challenge half marathon. I bagged a total of eight medals in six months.)

I ran the final marathon in this rush for medals, Los Angeles, in contemplation of mortality and with extreme gratitude for the chance to run again. I also ran with the assistance of guides to make sure my occasional vision and balance problems did not preclude me from finishing. It was a very different experience emotionally. I ran with different motives, in a different context, with a different basket of biases. To a large extent, the experience tempted me to reject or at least chafe against all I had learned up to that point. These truths were especially uncomfortable given my health and other challenges. In the case of my health problems, I wanted trial by combat. Driven by anger, I would find a way to triumph, emerging from the fight with the blood of my imagined enemy dripping from my hands and chin.

The possible diagnoses looming over my head each had their own clock and progression, but none of it was as good as not having a diagnosis looming over your head. I had decided to tell mortality and decay to fuck off: *I will show you I am not done. I am not weak. I may be going down, but I am going to rip a hole in the world on my way to the mat. I will kick the universe in the nuts and laugh. I will act, exercise my will in a significant way against everything that is ordained to happen to me. I will do so because I want to. I am not delusional. I know this will be the last futile gasp. Then, universe, I am all yours. Tear me apart, dissolve me painfully and slowly, but know this, March 8, 2020, I ran the LA Marathon! That was my day. I gave it to myself, and nothing can take it away from me. Take my hands. Take my legs. Kill me. I don't care. I already won. Fuck you.*

I wanted the last ounce of whatever I am to be a smear across the finish line. I wanted to use it all before it was taken.

I made a shirt for the marathon with the quotes always in my mind. I would wear my spirit, my will, my action. On the back of my shirt, it said, *I don't believe in the no-win scenario. —James T. Kirk* and *There are always possibilities. —Spock.*

On the front, in big letters, my shirt read, *To Strive, to Seek, to Find and* not *to Yield.*[25]

When running, I often played a favorite song called "Because I

---

25. This is the bitchin' boys' school, manly, nobody-can-stop-us stanza of a Tennyson poem about Ulysses.

Want to," written by a valued friend, the witty punk musician Fat Mike Burkett. A favorite verse:

> I'm gonna kick a hole.
> I'm gonna break a glass.
> I'm gonna fuck the world and kick its ass.

"Fuck the world and kick its ass." Indeed. That is how I lived for more than a year. The goal, the day—March 8, 2020—always in front of me. I could see everything. I would imagine how it would feel at the start, on every street, at every site, a course I could follow in my mind from start to finish. I had my family come out and my good friends meet me on the course. (Thank you!) I knew and planned for this being it. The end. The last time I would run. The last time I would be physically alive and capable. I was in the best shape of my life at age fifty-one, under my high-school wrestling weight, fit, motivated, focused. Angry.

This is tough to process and embarrassing to admit. In my fantasy world of rage, determination, and conflict (against whom, I did not need to know; the world, fate, physics?), I trained. I won. I would like to say all this reversion to anger was folly, but it was an awesome ride. I lived in violent fantasy, but this meant I got to be the star of my own movie every day. I was the hero, and I triumphed. Every day felt good. I had a purpose, no, a mission from the Fates, a destiny, like Luke staring toward the setting of Tatooine's binary suns. Every run was a victory. I would win. I even did the strength exercises that I hate on off days because my enemy was always at my heels, looking for any opening to strike. Every race felt like a step closer—Long Beach, Huntington Beach, Newport Beach, Santa Monica, Pasadena, and, finally my big day, the LA Marathon. I was never a struggling middle-aged runner. I was Harry at Agincourt. I was Kirk retaking the

---

and tho'
We are not now that strength which in old days
Moved earth and heaven, that which we are, we are;
One equal temper of heroic hearts,
Made weak by time and fate, but strong in will
To strive, to seek, to find, and not to yield.

Enterprise from Khan. I was going over the top at Gallipoli. I was Jack Aubrey slashing my way to the enemy quarterdeck. (I am good at fantasy.) I was living everywhere but reality. This was so much better than reality. I was screaming down this ill-advised path precisely because I was unhappy with reality, and I felt reality gifted me a window to do something outside it. When my big, final test arrived, I was grateful to share it with my guides, lovely young people who I am sure were disappointed they got me and not a blind guy. I saw my family, parents, and the few friends who have been with me for the whole ride. Members of the Achilles running club, the group that helped me out with guides, came up to say hello. I love this course, this city. So many of the things I love are on the route. Much of my life that I can peg to one place or another is part of the course. There was no cataclysmic breakdown, but it was not an easy run. It hurt, and I worked very hard to stay under fifteen minutes per mile. (Don't laugh unless you know the effort and pain that time required.) I am sure it looked beyond ugly. Occasionally I would really run hard for a few yards to demonstrate that I could, but there was a long and heavy price to be paid thereafter. Ultimately, the first ocean breeze, a turn down Ocean Boulevard, and the finish just a mile ahead. By this point, I was crying and laughing, as alive and fulfilled as I would ever be. My efforts to really run to the finish never made it more than a few steps, but I found it for the last fifty yards. I expected this to be the last finish line I would cross, the last time I would run like this, and I wanted to leave it all on the course. I ran hard, pumping my arms as if I were running the 440 in a high-school track meet. If I could have ended everything there, if I had a button I could push that would turn my body into a smear of blood across the finish line, I would have pushed it. If I had an option to die like Pheidippides upon crossing the line, I would have taken it, though something more Michael Bay with explosions would have matched my emotions better. I leaped and shouted as I went over the timing strip, conscious of what the photo would look like but completely sincere too. I stumbled into some fencing and then was pushed farther into the chute by someone. Complete and total vindication and victory. I was in so much pain but grinning and laughing from pure giddiness. This was absolute, unadulterated triumph. Someone should have been following me, whispering in my ear, "Remember thou art mortal."

The run and leap at the end had cost me dearly, but I had not only seen the top of the mountain, I was there. Truly, if that could have been my end, if you asked me right now if I would like to finish life in that moment, without hesitation, I would answer yes. It was glorious. I was happy.

So all my thinking, all my close observation, all my practice and learning, all jettisoned in exchange for angry fantasy. My first major test having believed I had cracked the code for human contentment, and I revert to the negative states I rejected.

I was not in reality. I was never doing what I really was doing. I chose not to train for and run in a race. I made training and racing a means to prove to myself and the universe that I was better than I feared. My medical problems and difficulties had a personality, a monster that could be fought, insidious malware. My problems were imposed on me by someone, a villain in my story. That villain had some agenda in attacking me, cared about the outcome, was watching my progress and rooting against me. There was someone I wanted to prove something to, and he would be watching, furious that I had frustrated his plans for me. Nonsense on stilts wrapped in gibberish. None of these fancies had a lot to do with the realities. There were medical problems, maybe neurochemical, genetic, but just medical problems that happen, chemistry that happens without a knowing, vengeful wizard or Bond villain making it happen. There was a desire to train to move my body over a distance in a specified time on a specific date. That is it. Some medical problems. Training for a run. When a physical problem is big, unsettling, and may end in death or something else quite bad, it is easy to shift to fantasy and anger, make life a fight to be won. You hear this all the time. He "fought" cancer. I was not immune.

I jettisoned reality for a life in angry fantasy. I cannot deny how good it felt. I cannot deny how it got me through training to goals that an objective, more sedate, and thoughtful approach would have probably rejected altogether. March 8, 2020, really was the day I wanted it to be. Part of me still feels like I fucked the world and kicked its ass that day. No. All of me does. I won. The universe lost. Those are the emotions.

However, my permanent address is in reality even if I vacation in violent boys' fantasies. I am left with pain, an inability to exercise as I would like, and the psychic, mood, and physical costs of that. My year of running dangerously no matter the cost ended with two back surgeries within a year, and I truly may have traded one glorious day at the LA Marathon for a lifetime of pain and some debility. I had constructed this fantasy to make this race my final triumphant shout into the night, yelling, "Blow, winds, and crack your cheeks! Rage!" like Lear or riding my motorcycle into the night around Dead Man's Curve. It made for great fantasy, but now it is over. Now I really do not want that to be the last time I run, and it does not have to be. Being Robin Hood shooting a final arrow through the window of his hospital room in Kirklees Priory, telling Little John to bury him where it lands, well, that is a bigger, more seductive life than "Let's focus on rebuilding core strength and dropping weight."

In taking this path of violent fantasy so contrary to what I had discovered to be true, I ended up validating, yet again, the things I had already learned. I arrived again at the conclusion that however one may feel or want the world to be, it is the way it is.

You Can Only Finish in the Real World

Internal denial or ignorance is blindness or delusion. One path, reality, leads to finishing . . . possibly. The road of delusion leads to pain and failure . . . ultimately, certainly.

I know the allure of anger and fantasies of conflict. I know the seductive short-term pop they offer. They must be fought. This is a great, necessary discipline. Keep your objective mind and what you know is actually true at the fore and follow it. Reject the temporary ecstasy of the drug. The Siren call of a fight is always there. Take on rejecting that call as an active, conscious discipline on the path.

I had the knowledge. I had not adequately developed the discipline to resist the temptation that awaited me when I thought my window for living was closing, and when it called, I failed.

The feeling and motivation that led to such short-term success rested on a fantasy that there is a universe that watches or cares. There is not. There is no drama between you and your cancer any more than there is drama between you and gravity when you fall. We want our misfortune to be part of a movie, but there just is not a script in the multiplication of cells or having someone crash into you.

Now living in reality, I cannot run, and managing pain is a major feature of my life. I beg my doctors for pain pills. I drink to find peace. I am prone to negative cycles of depression, more things to fight off. Not wise.

Pain Is the Great Test of Discipline

In *The Heart of the Buddha's Teaching*, Thích Nhất Hạnh offers a life lesson: "Don't throw away your suffering. Touch your suffering. Face it directly, and your joy will become deeper."

Pain is unavoidable. You will live with pain, maybe all the time. You are decaying and will die. This means pain. For some, pain is the greatest test of the discipline to pursue happiness, because the presence of certain pain may put "happiness" in any conventional sense out of reach.

Pain is a condition of the mind but very real and can be debilitating. It would be facile, counterfactual, and useless to say it is all in your head. Therefore, if you control your mind, you are in control of pain. Bull fucking shit. Perhaps there have been some ascended masters who could be indifferent to having their face set on fire. Perhaps. That does not matter. Pain hurts. It is unpleasant. Maybe it is terrible and unbearable. Maybe it is slow, grinding pain. Everything in my worldview is premised on seeing things clearly as they really are. Pain is a fact. Pain is inevitable. Many of us will die with a morphine button in our hand because there is nothing left before the grave but pain.

Usually, pain poses no more problem to finding joy than any other unpleasant obstacle. We can deal with it because we know it is transitory. The agony of the broken leg will pass. The subtler persistent pain that follows will fade in days. You know that in weeks you should be at this stage of healing, at months here, and so on. It is really just a detour, something to get through. We put pain outside our journey, something in the way that will pass, just a source of nuisance and delay. As a result, we do not usually really have to recognize pain as part of our lives, and we do not. Pain is an aberration.

This view of pain as an unlucky thing that is outside our lives ignores the fact of pain. It is taking a big part of life and cutting it out because it makes the rest of the time happier. It is cutting out a rotten chunk of the apple and then saying the apple is great through and through. Maybe you acknowledge that there was a rot problem, but you pushed on and got through it. That is my father's approach. His choice to be happy is really a choice to deny, avoid, or discount pain. This move does not work when you face persistent pain with no realistic hope of relief soon enough for you to hold fast. If you have spinal cord damage or have cancer eating away at your brain, you have pain, all the time. If you exclude pain as part of your life, you have no life.

You must find joy through a radical conciliation with your pain. You must choose to love your path, pain included. You cannot merely endure pain. You must find a way to live with it and go forward productively. This is a matter of discipline and a real test. This may be "the" test in life.

If pain is an unpleasant waiting room where you watch the clock until the receptionist tells you your life may continue, you will die in the waiting room.

True reconciliation with pain may not be possible because we are not all transcendent Zen masters and yogis. One of the great joys of running and other physically challenging endeavors is you get to play with pain. You get to see what you can do working with pain. For someone like me, there are hours in a marathon where it seems there is nothing else but pain, even consciousness falls away into something that feels much less personal. It is just me and my pain, testing my discipline to control my body and achieve my goal. This, however, is merely play. I know the race will end and, with it, the significant pain. I know I can quit and the pain will quit. The test is whether or not I choose to end the pain by quitting. That is nothing like the test of chronic pain or pain from a disease. You do not get to take a walk, drink some Gatorade, and decide if you can go in for another round of pain. Running is useful, but it is merely a simulator when it comes to the real discipline of pain.

It would be glib to say every life is worth living all the time regard-less of pain. Nurses in hospice do not, I hope, tell patients, "Tough it out, just rub some dirt on it. You'll be feeling great tomorrow." When life runs into its only inevitability, it is hard to acknowledge what is happening, that this is life, that this life exists largely to feel terrible pain, and the only respite will be death. Fantasies get us through the waiting room and back into action! Life is for the living and so on. It is easy to fall back on fantasies of anger and conflict, to view things happening as a fight most strongly perhaps when there is no fight, just a very unpleasant reality—pain. It is not just the patient who wants the cancer to be a personified bad guy. We want the guy in pain who will be dead in three months to be a warrior fighting the bad guy because we do not want to observe and accept what is really happening to our friend, our wife, a fellow human. Because we know what is happening will happen to us, we want to pretend that it is not happening. Fantasy is an alluring and powerful motivation, but even in the fantasy, the sick person suffers and dies. You cannot outlive reality.

Pain is tough to watch. Surviving loved ones look at the last days of a person that were dominated by pain as a tragedy, and the sooner death ended things, the better. We would take death over pain. We would take death over seeing pain. That is true for everyone whatever you say now. Even if pain may not go on forever, everyone has a break-ing point. If you are not leading an examined life, it may all seem un-fair. You may live, but you may do so in anger and disbelief of what is happening. For those who recognize the reality of pain, discipline will eventually fail. If the end of pain is death, if there really is no cake and ice cream waiting for us, if we just hang in longer, death does not seem like a solution or comfort, just an end. Just hanging in for any end, even with treatment and a likely end of pain, may not be a realis-tic option. What matters is having the discipline to persist until pain ends or is otherwise managed. I can make no judgment on someone who cannot embrace their pain. How much torture could I endure? How soon would the end have to be to support me through the ordeal? How likely would that end have to be? I do not know. I hope I do not find out. I make no judgment on how anyone answers those questions. Before that point when the negative experience of pain is greater than life, I hope to continue to find ways to embrace my pain.

You can train for pain. There are some Buddhist traditions that view the whole of life as preparing for our final breath.[26] Former POWs and Holocaust survivors tend to write very good books. Their experiences were terrible, and I am sure they felt entirely hopeless. Having seen what they have seen, faced what they have faced, they were forced to live—observe, analyze, and figure out how to respond to—circumstances where the consequences were life and death, rotting away or torture, or maybe even reward for acting badly. As I bang away on my keyboard in my backyard, by the pool, living the life of permanent vacation, I know that those who have been to hell and back have had experiences and the opportunity to accrue wisdom that I will not have. I have no privileged perspective here.

The period following my final run, the LA Marathon, the year after my ill-advised quest through fantasy to run my body into nothingness, was a dive into pain. It was really the first time I was forced to accept pain as an enduring part of my reality. Cysts and fluid in a vertebra were pressing on the sciatic nerve. To make life more interesting, the channels out of which the nerve exits the vertebra were collapsing as a result of arthritis. I went through a lot of medicine with no diagnosis, a lot of physical therapy resulting in an increase in pain. I had no hope, just a life of pain before me.

I had surgery to remove the cysts and the lamina (the sheet of bone on the back of the vertebra) in order to relieve fluid pressure. That pain vanished.

I was not wholly unprepared for the experience. The work I had done, intentional and not necessarily fun life work, got me through long enough for my path to cross with the right surgeon's. My life with the pain was not good. There was no relief. I did not really sleep much without the aid of drugs, exhaustion, dozing off, waking with a yell as I'd get a new shot of pain, repeat. I wanted out. What is the point of being alive if your primary function is to be a thing that suffers? I spent a lot of time contemplating this. How could evolution end up producing creatures that just suffer, whose suffering could be their only function and experience? The answer, I think, lies in the nasty, brutish, and

---

26. For the teacher, this has the same benefit as the Christian heaven—nobody is alive to say if you are wrong.

short nature of the real world. I have outlived my usefulness and would not suffer because I should have been crushed by a mastodon years ago, giving way to younger, more able men in the social grouping. This makes the logic of ending life all the more powerful. Not only do I want to be dead to end the pain but, really, the pain is telling me that I should be dead. I am past my expiration date.

Training for Pain

I went into this experience equipped with a mind better able to manage pain through training. If I did not want to stay for myself, I wanted to stay for my family. I could live and do so marching toward important goals if not for my own pleasure in the conventional sense, then as a meaningful part of the lives of others. I learned this move through my psychiatric existential crises. There was the hard-nosed therapist who said whatever I may think of myself or life or anything else, my actions could be disastrous for my children. Reality. So I knew the move—get outside myself. How does this impact others I want to help? It's a strong move.

I also had experience with pain and some understanding of how to process pain—pain in life, in sports, and particularly in play. I could anticipate the negative thoughts and feelings I would package around pain, and I knew how to manage them both—the pain as well as the unhelpful thoughts and feelings I injected into the scenario. I also had some confidence because, at least in the short run, I knew how I would fare managing them. I knew what it was like to go deep into pain and be isolated alone with pain—Chicago Marathon. I knew that if you give yourself a chance, unexpectedly good results may flow—Los Angeles Marathon. I did not have to be afraid of anything. I know how to live with pain, even if there is no coming out on the other side at the finish.

An examined life that takes you on purposeful simulations of the pain you will experience will give you greater wisdom, better tactics, and greater confidence for the road ahead. There is some payoff for the metaphorical training and simulations on all the metaphorical race days up to the point of decision. One can seek out experiences like running that are a simple and potentially extreme test bed. Running has been my sandbox, but anything that taxes the body in a controlled way without great consequences for failure is a useful thing to have in one's life. My father could not understand why I would spend my time toying with the purposeful infliction of pain. He did not accept pain as a part of life, and we need to find contentment with it where I found it interesting and in a way pleasurable. In the vicissitudes and struggles of pain, without preparation, a person would likely be reduced to something entirely reactive and entirely suffering without any preparation.

When it is not a simulation that you can end or modify, one should still look at experiences with pain as objects of study. Life itself is iterative, each iteration a simulation for the next. Consistent and hopefully ultimately continuous practice of mindfulness, that is, careful observation of what is happening, makes ordinary life and experience itself an object of study, present life a training exercise for the future. Running and sitting and climbing, even though pursued for the purpose of examining pain and other challenges are part of the practitioner's life as well. However, when one has the choice to end the pain, the psychological challenge is much lighter.

So much about watching my father's death was instructive. He was unprepared for the pain, and the pain coupled with a decline in mental capacity was not pretty. Suffering was etched into his destiny. He was human. He would have great pain, but his suffering was so very sad, like seeing a confused, wounded animal, just suffering, nothing else, just suffering. He could not just choose to be happy and be happy. His easygoing life overlooked choices he could have made that would have made the end of his life better.

Happiness itself is not within one's control per se, but it is within our power to lighten the experience of pain and create the conditions for happiness with things we can accomplish in our minds. You can train for this.

Why Choose a "Happiness" That Includes Pain?

Medical and physical therapy may lead to improvement on improvement or greater and greater accommodation of pain. Often recovery tracks a logarithmic hockey-stick curve, a slow slog at the beginning and improvement on improvement on the way to the starting line. Each diminishment of pain, the physical feeling, and the psychic benefit of seeing improvement make it easier at each succeeding decision point to choose happiness even with pain and even with the added work of trying to diminish the pain.

It's important to feel good about what you have done. At age one hundred, my grandmother-in-law exercised with a hand cycle that physical therapists brought in. Her body was withered, but the joy and pride in her eyes and smile were that of sixteen-year-old Berta back in Swabia circa 1916, showing her mates exactly how it's done in the gym. There was not any hint of irony or disappointment or acknowledgment that it might not be a big deal to someone else. One hundred. Pride in growing and showing strength. There are no light weights. There are no slow times. I wish I could thank her for that moment. I had no idea that that moment would mean anything in my life. Eighteen years later, I understand, and I am grateful.

I notice this when recovering from surgery, going from total incapacity, needing someone to hold the plastic jug while you pee in bed, to getting out and about again. It happens rapidly for most things, in mere weeks. The early accomplishments—getting out of bed, peeing by yourself, walking to the mailbox—these are major achievements. I have not been able to do x, and not doing x is something I notice frequently. It may even be a source of humiliation. When you can do x, it is a moment. When I run, each incremental improvement drives me to the next. Starting from a point of obesity, getting that first mile was huge. I did it! I want more. Two miles! I can't believe I am doing this! I have never gone this far before. I did not think I would ever run this far . . .

The same is true of the mental, contemplative work that can drastically reduce the subjective experience of pain. The tangible improvements are motivating, elevating, and generally fantastic. Many who practice meditation chase the dragon of calmness, emptiness. They had a good sit (meditation session), felt open and relaxed, de-stressed, and they want that feeling to be their lives. That is great, but chasing pain relief is even better. Equanimity is something for people who can sit down without shouting in pain. Pain has some gifts. It is a wonderful object of study, and if you can sit with it—the nature of it, the experience of it, watching it expand and contract—it provides problems and extremes that make it a great laboratory. If you are healthy, seek pain. It has much more to teach than simple pleasure and as such offers its own more complex variety of pleasure. Pain is a more sensitive and easier-to-read gauge than contentment. The reward of relieving pain is wonderful, liberating, effectively a shot of physical pleasure. Finding balance in sensation is a minuet. Relieving pain is a rave. A nice lie-down versus sex. Living in pain and the abatement of that pain in any degree is a joy and inspiration to keep going, observing, learning, thinking until the pain is the smallest thing it can be in your life.

Pain is a part of your life. You do not have a choice. It may come to dominate every moment. You must embrace it as a part of your life, not a time-out, something to wait out, get past so your life can resume. It is a necessary dimension of our existence. If you hold pain as something alien to be endured or dispatched so you can move on, you are missing out on your actual life. Considering periods dominated by pain as something outside of regulation play takes those periods away from you. That outlook also cuts your life short. If you consider pain as something that stands in the way of your life, and if pain is an inescapable reality in your life, your life is over. The years you spend in pain will be unnecessarily unhappy. You will be angry. You will feel that pain has robbed you unfairly of your time. It is exactly the opposite, you have robbed yourself by refusing to accept your actual situation, your actual life.

Pain is terrible. It is not easy. However, you cannot hide from pain. You must live within it. It is the test we may not face until our final days, but the test will likely come. Pain could end your life. Maybe the unpleasantness taxes your discipline too heavily, maybe it intrudes on everything else too much for you to make it forward in life. However, radically accepting pain as part of your circumstance makes going forward and doing so if not with a smile, then with an ease and openness, possible. You can choose a happiness that includes pain. If you do, the pain is less damaging; wise action is possible; accurate and useful observations and thought will follow; and things will likely get better even if they will never be good.

CHAPTER 17

Choose Happiness Right Now

We have the present, this moment, right now. The future may offer nothing but pain and death. (Spoiler alert, it almost certainly does.) The past may be a pit of failure as deep as the Mariana Trench, making an escape seem impossible. Yet here we are, not in an imagined future or a remembered past, both things in fantasy and likely magnified by whatever fears and insecurities lurk in our outlook. We are here. We are not fully content and wish to be happier. The choice to be happy must be made now. That choice is a necessary first step that must precede all others. If you wish to be happy, if you wish to find contentment, to move forward, to live any kind of purposeful life, and not just drift or be pushed and pulled by often negative forces, you must choose happiness right now. Everything is contingent on that choice.

I spent a lot of time lying in bed next to my father in his final days. I told his stories. His verbal responses turned to smiles turned to a squeeze of the hand turned to listening, but I know he was hearing and understanding up to maybe his final eight hours. I told family stories from my own time, my brother getting trapped outside SeaWorld when everyone else was inside; the time my other brother trapped himself in my grandmother's bathroom and my father had to climb through the window to retrieve him, my grandmother screaming as if the building were collapsing. I told stories from my family that predate me but I know are true, how excited he was to have met my mother in Cincinnati at a fraternity convention and his decision to cancel interviewing at business schools to fly back to her. (Was this real life or a Hugh Grant movie?) I told his childhood stories, how he and his best friend, Johnny, sneaked into a hotel to get Joe DiMaggio's autograph, managed to get to the slugger's room, knocked on the door, and returned with the autograph. Our family was nuts in often hilarious ways. There is a reason so many comedians and comedy writers are Jews. Mel Brooks and Jerry Seinfeld are storytellers not novelists. My family fit a lot of the comic molds. My family was bananas. Ups, downs, love, loss, birth, death, all of it, but my father had a good life, and he was not at all off the mark to have loved it.[27]

I had a lot of time to think about the path that brought each of us to that moment, a dying father and a son who had struggled to live despite having every advantage. So different, each with such a different experience and view, yet we were there in the same moment. The thoughts ran to this writing. My father was the only person who had read any of it. He believed it had value for me, and it made him proud as a father. This would be a positive way he would live on. He was

---

27. The unstated, but always felt black vacuum behind all this is the Holocaust. (This is not ancient history. This is my parents.) My parents were permitted to live, date, enjoy the *Happy Days* life, have a family in a ranch house amid lemon trees and mountains, and have me because some maverick left home in the 1880s for America. Blind luck. Whoever, whatever was in Europe is unknown, unremembered, and definitely not discussed. Gone. Dying in Upland, California, seventy years later in an adjustable bed, with an American passport in the drawer and UCLA yearbooks on the shelf—what an extraordinary gift. He never said anything, but it had to be on his mind always. After hanging in high school with Potsie and the gang, he returned to a home hosting Jewish refugees. There was total awareness and appreciation. When I was younger and burned with outrage at social injustice, I was angry at my father for his complacency. I view him differently now. He understood and loved what he had. He did not need more and would never ask for more.

surprised he had an impact on me even if not in the typical way. We always stared at each other over a gulf of incomprehension, but our root failures were the same, just viewed from different directions.

The Sins of the Father: Choosing Happiness Despite the Future

Watching my father die was unpleasant, not so much for the illness and the end in death per se, but my father's inability truly up to the end to view his illness and death as something that would or should happen. He was not an idiot. He was an intelligent man, a practical businessperson and lawyer, with it, complete, smart, not delusional. He understood what was happening. The doctors, then the hospice nurse, confirmed the obvious at every step. If you asked him what was going on inside him, he could tell you all about the metastatic cancer, the course of treatment, its end, and his prognosis. He knew he was dying and was more interested in giving me tour after tour of his financial records and directions on how to handle taxes postmortem than telling tales. He was not delusional.

At the same time, he never really accepted what was happening. It all seemed a terrible, unexpected, undeserved unfairness. He was eighty. He had months of notice of his death and was really pain free with the aid of drugs up until his final days. He was robust and in full capacity up until his final days. There was no tragedy that I could see. This is how it happens *if* we are fortunate. This is life. This is a good life. Even my father with all his affability and laid-back comfort with the world was not immune. Nobody is. He was going to die and undergo the experience of decay and death. It would hurt. A lot. It did.

He had always chosen happiness, which, for him, meant ignoring the negative. This does not lead to any sort of profound contentment or understanding, but it is a fine way to just enjoy the day. He could no longer do this. For the first time in his life, he encountered something unpleasant he could not simply whistle past or turn his back on and let pass. This could not be ignored. He was going to die. He would have increasing pain to the point of screaming and begging for death. He did.

He could not choose to be happy as he had before.

His teeth were black. His arteries visible through tissue-paper skin as a dark-gray honeycomb lattice. He knew he had bouts of moody insanity. Yet when the hospice nurse told him perhaps four days before his death that the dying process had begun, my father was distraught. He still seemed to think that there was something unfair or unexpected. It seemed bizarre to me. What did he think was happening? He knew, but he did not accept the truth of what was known at the same time.

A reflective person knows this is always a possibility. My father had to confront this truth about six months before his death, upon being read the writ of execution from his doctor onward. To be happy, he would have to choose to be happy knowing that the immediate future was rough and short. He never had to do this. This, to me, was the sad aspect of his death.

There is the tragedy of time wasted. He had about six months of full capacity. It could have been a productive and beautiful time for him. He had his children around him for the first time in roughly twenty years. Petty disagreements were put on hold. He had motivation to say and do everything that had been put off, talk to friends, partake in new experiences, revel in memories, pass on whatever he thought he had to give. There was no bucket list. There was not even scheduling quality time with the people he cared about. When an old friend or relative called, he was thrown into a fit of sadness and despair. He knew the call was a goodbye, and he did not want to say goodbye. He cried all the time. He had to be distracted from his life.

Given my bent for extremes, I offered everything I could get for him, from a tour of his old fraternity house to ketamine with Thai ladyboys and anything else he fancied. He never was interested in adding something to his life that was not already there. Thinking of things to do to be happy and then doing them was just not part of his life. He never had any desire to travel before his impending doom—why would he now? He could have labeled old pictures so the family albums would not be discarded upon his death. It could have been the biggest six months of his life. It could have represented a level of contentment, joy, and understanding that outweighed the prior forty years. No. He relied upon his move—ignore the negative, and then everything is positive.

In the end, looking at the reality of death, he could not choose to be happy and simply be happy. The present was pain, and the future was death. Ignoring the negative left him with very little.

By refusing to accept and work within the reality of the situation, he lost the gift of his last six months.

By refusing to choose happiness with positive action, to take steps to engender happiness, there was nothing in his life likely to make him happy.

He never had to think, accept, or act. By persisting in his sunny-side-of-the-street mode of living, he made his final days ones of terror and disbelief. He never let go of life. He held on tight and watched reality slowly saw his hands off at the wrist.

It was difficult to witness. Ultimately, he had nothing but suffering. He could not speak, but whenever the nurse moved him, his face contorted in an effort to scream. He was beyond screaming. There was no counterbalancing force of gratitude or ease when the immediate torment subsided.

He wasted what time he had. He died in agony and terror.

His death will always be a source of pain and guilt for those around him. We watched him suffer and die, impotent, as he cried for help.

In a way, David Grossman presents the problem of the lotus eater. He had his drug—a self-made ability to ignore the unpleasant and focus on the things that supported his happiness. He was able to live in fantasy. In the end, and I am sure at points along the way, reality tore down the pleasant facades he constructed. I am sure he could not always drive down Skid Row and see only the bits that would compose something like Main Street at Disneyland, overlooking the squalor and poverty so only the gorgeous Art Deco and Mediterranean architecture behind the filth remained. However, he could always get back to the happiness he chose, until he could not. Reality ultimately won.

He was unable to choose a happiness that included pain. Along the way, throughout his entire life, he missed so much of the world. He shortchanged himself on finding joy in the body and mind. He never approached the higher joys of contentment and equanimity. A world in which you can choose to be happy without observation, thought, or discipline has to be a simple one, one far simpler than reality. If you can simply choose to be happy, your happiness cannot be anything that requires the development of knowledge or taste. It cannot be anything that is challenging, anything that includes any level of discomfort. Such magical choice can exist only in fantasy, and that world of fantasy has to be small and familiar. I hope he was happy in life. I think he was, even if he passed up many opportunities as the cost of closing his eyes as he whistled past the graveyard. I certainly always envied how he and the world seemed so copacetic. If given the choice to live in his skin, most of the time, I would do so. If given the choice to take the parts of the world that were nice and leave the rest outside my view, often I would take my father's path. However, as with drugs, ignorance, and anything else that eschews present reality, you will crash against reality, and there is so much reality has to offer.

I wish he did not suffer so.

I wish I could have shared so many things with him that just were not a part of his world. He was always perplexed at my desire to run. I would try to explain how contentment lies in the difficulty of training and how the singular experience of being alone with nothing but your pain and desire at mile eighteen is a pinnacle of existence. He could not understand. He knew I read and I had a rich internal life, but that probably seemed like work in the one case and escape from a good life in the other. Why would you dress up in costumes and live in a shared fantasy? He had some understanding that I pursued sense pleasures outside the norm, but they remained unacknowledged. We never talked about the agony in the orgasm, not even close. Again, why would you want to reach the heights of imagination? Of physical possibility? Why would you support an identity with pain and accomplishment? Why would you seek experience so far outside your normal life?

In the big picture, why would you be unhappy even as part of some program for a greater or different happiness later? Why look for pleasures not at hand? It does not make sense; just be happy. He had never had present pain or a grim prognosis. When he did, everything failed.

I am grateful we had our trip to Yellowstone. That conversation, which continues today in my mind, provokes me. He was a decent man, the only one I have ever met. I am not. He was naturally happy. I am not. How he had me as a son is a puzzle for the universe.

Maybe we understood each other better at the end.

The Sins of the Son: Choosing
Happiness Despite the Past

My father may have missed out on a lot, and his final months may have been squandered in apathy and terror. However, his "always look on the bright side of life" way of moving through the world supported 79.5 years of a *Candide*-level optimism in exchange for a rough few months at the end that could have been great.[28] He lived in his own Elysium: Upland, California. I have lived in far greater sin, a far greater waste of life. I have spent years, probably most of my life, living outside the actual occurrence of events by dwelling in the past. If you are in the past, you cannot choose to pursue happiness in the present.

Every imperfect thing I ever said, every person who did not like me, every tiny embarrassment, it all continues, bile to be regurgitated ad infinitum. I still wince when I recall failures from childhood. I have to focus and use the various intellectual techniques I have to return to what is happening and see a memory for what it is, almost nothing arising from a world that no longer exists, having no practical impact on anything I am doing and existing solely as an image in my mind. Tamping down prior failures and regret remains work. I do not fear an unpleasant future as my father did. For me, choosing to pursue happiness is conscious work to leave the past.

There is a great old *Twilight Zone* episode, "The Sixteen-Millimeter Shrine," in which a glamorous star of the silver screen cannot manage the reality of her aging and all the loss that comes with it. She lives alone in her mansion, curtains shutting out the Beverly Hills sunshine, watching and rewatching her old films, lost in a world that has passed but is still available to see as reflected light on a screen. Ultimately, her rejection of reality becomes so great that she reenters the screen. She enters the physical screen in her screening room and actually becomes a part of the film being shown, living forever as she wished to be, young, glamorous, famous, surrounded by chivalrous and dashing gentlemen, locked in the stories recorded on film. Fantasy.

Rod Serling surely intended to hold out the Norma Desmond

---

28. My father's game plan is much easier for someone with material comfort and health than others.

character as someone deeply delusional and self-destructive. Ultimately, she lost all grasp of reality or understood reality too well and opted for fantasy. However, she wanted to be someplace great, a movie star playing princesses and lovers. I was not so smart.

I spent much of my life between ages thirty-nine and fifty lying in bed, often awake, staring at the ceiling, lost in a cyclone of memories, emotions, and analytical thought, all different expressions of how much I hated myself, how much I regretted what had happened and how my decisions have impacted my family negatively. I lost years. At least the Norma Desmond character and my father chose a positive fantasy; I opted for living in a motion picture of self-hatred and misery.

Even though the movie on the ceiling was a tragedy, it was a comfortable place for me to hide. The psychological masochism of brooding over old failures is comfortable for me, my natural way. Beating myself up is the old pair of jeans you have been wearing so long the fabric is stretched to a perfect mold of your body.

At one particularly dark stage, I had quit my job and, with my dysfunction, foisted a great deal of stress on my wife and confusion and insecurity on my young children. If it all needed comic expression, as we were managing our effective eviction, we had a flood that made the first story of our house uninhabitable and filled it with loud fans and workers cutting out drywall. Our furniture and things were already reduced to jumbled piles. I winced with each tick of the clock, seeing no solution short of stopping time. It was all coming apart. I had nowhere to go, nothing I could do. The only good thing in my life was two million dollars in life insurance. The things I could and should have been doing were not a mystery—talk to people, get my name out, etc.—but the enormity of my failures kept me from doing anything. I could not get past them.

I would help get my kids off to school, help pick them up, but otherwise I was lying in bed, staring at the ceiling, wanting out, guilty for creating the situation, trying to convince myself that my children would be better off without a father if the father had to be me, panicked as I could feel time passing and the problems growing. With each moment, I hated myself even more because another moment had passed and I had done nothing to make things better.

My perspective was beyond distorted, Dr. Caligari's cabinet within a stucco house in Carmel Valley, California. I generally was focused on meta, strategic problems, and that was all I could see. In that scope, anything I could actually do in the moment was pointless. My prior failures were so enormous that the story of the future was already written.

A business phrase popular at the time comes to mind. Anything I did would be rearranging deck chairs on the *Titanic*. There was nothing to do but wait for the splash.

I had the intellectual gifts to move forward for sure. My success in law and business has generally been about playing failure into profit, jujitsu via bankruptcy reorganization, creative asset sale, corporate structure, or complex licensing scheme. I was creative, comfortable in first-of-a-kind situations and one-of-a-kind situations and generally good at it. However, that is what I did for other people. I viewed my simpler situation as being truly hopeless. Like Kirk said to his adult son (who for some reason we did not know about for the first twenty-five years of the son's life), "I haven't faced death. [A very manly fellow exposes himself.] I've cheated death. [He pauses to consider his life and how he has an adult son he does not even recognize.] I've tricked my way out of death and patted myself on the back for my ingenuity. [He knows he is the Odysseus of the galaxy; he confesses the inescapable conclusion.] I know nothing . . . [of death.]" This was it. My Kobayashi Maru for my Trekker friends.[29] It was over.

My situation was hopeless because I had defined the conditions of my life exam to be hopeless, keeping the enormity of all prior mistakes with me in every moment. Like young James Tiberius understood, the

---

29. For those of you too culturally deprived to know *Star Trek II: The Wrath of Khan*, STII:TWOK if you want to sound like you know geeky things, the Kobayashi Maru is a test given to Starfleet cadets. It is a simulation in which the student playing captain of a Starfleet ship is placed in an impossible situation. Every decision leads to the death of many people. There is no solution. The purpose of the test is to learn what it is like to be in a no-win scenario. Of course, one student, a young James Tiberius Kirk, rejects the notion of a no-win scenario and was the only cadet ever to pass the exam. He reprogrammed the computer so the problem could be solved. I generally agree with Kirk. Short of death, I don't believe in the no-win scenario. The challenge in life is to define the parameters of any challenge so success is possible. It is not cheating. It is surviving.

solution lies in changing the parameters of the test so that there is a solution. I did not choose to pursue happiness. I did not think the choice was before me. As a result, I did not do the many obvious things I could do to move forward. Perhaps that is why I was not offered a starship command in my thirties.

In writing this, I realized that when I was staring at the ceiling throughout that decade, I was not just hating myself and rehashing all the existing reasons I did. I really was stuck in a specific moment I could not get past. As I stared at the ceiling year after year, and any time I want to torment myself even now, I replay the night of my significant overdose. I have strobed slices of that night as I went in and out of consciousness, but those flashbulb images are clear, as are the thought and emotion tied to each. It is all vivid, tangible, more like present perception than memory. Lucid. Undiminished by time. I do not know today's date or whether I did the thing I just did, but I remember everything about that night. It was a lot of life crammed into a few hours.

For forty years I fantasized about finally graduating from suffering. For a brief time, it felt like I had finally won. I felt free. I remember the sense of hustle, the flash of paramedics putting me into a wheelchair. I was no longer afraid. I was happy. I finally did what I knew had to be done since I was a toddler. Then I was on a table, and a nurse kept slapping me. I saw my wife. The pain I had caused her was plain. I opened my eyes again, and my parents were standing there. In hindsight, this may have been a hallucination, but my memory is clear. And always there was an officious nurse politely calling me "Mr. Grossman" while slapping me, screaming at me, people moving me around to clean the shit that I was leaking everywhere.

I had enough clarity to understand where I was and know that I had failed. I was alive and ashamed and angry at myself for it. I had shat the bed figuratively and literally. It was hopeless. I would live.

When I was on my bed at home in the decade that followed, I was not really on my bed. When I was looking at the ceiling, I was not really looking at the ceiling. I was on the table in the hospital. I was watching a screen capturing the crisp Technicolor projections of my mind that night. I was reliving every moment in the event and every motivation and thought leading up to it and every regret and recrimination after it. My present reality was laden with every error of the past that ran from childhood all the way up to "to be or not to be." Every moment was pregnant with decision and a bare bodkin pressed against my jugular. I was forever splicing each phrase of Hamlet's soliloquy with images of my own life and the palpable feelings attached to them.

I was stuck, in a purgatory. I did not live in the present. I was not where I was. I was a ghost roaming my own house, looking at my family from some distant remove, like a spirit of failed suburban dad past.

I was not sure I wanted to live. I was not sure I wanted to die either. I relived that experience, the mistakes I made in the execution of my plan, whether I could have played it differently in the hospital so that I did die. Was my continued life a choice? Was it cowardice, wisdom, or an excuse? I had caused and continued to cause such harm to my family. Was the night in the hospital a rebirth or a botched execution? The whole episode seemed childish and beneath me, a Wile E. Coyote, Rube Goldberg plan that belied a lack of real intent. The shame of it expressed in the harm to my family was just overwhelming. At least the prince of Denmark limits his vacillation to about six hours on stage. I went on for a decade and extend it further with this writing.

As I was living in the movie on the ceiling, my entire life ended on that hospital table. All that came before was important only as a step on the forever ineluctable path to the table. All memory was viewed from the wrong end of the telescope. I was almost always distracted, physically present, but not seeing the reality in which I lived as having any importance. So pointless and destructive in a quiet, painfully-rotting-out-from-the-center sort of way.

All I could see in the present was the damage I had done. The noise of the fans drying out the walls and the workmen downstairs told me in every moment that I had broken the stability of our family and we were losing our home because of me. The happy voices and laughter of my children hurt. My boundless love for them translated directly into my self-hatred for how I had hurt them and would continue to hurt them through the future with the ongoing echoes of my failures. I wondered who would be the person to tell me to get out of bed and leave, that this was not my beautiful house and that this was not my beautiful wife and this was not my life. Each mistake and each consequence were etched into cement that could only grow harder and more intractable with each tick and tock. The present and future existed solely to etch the past into stone tablets.

Given the enormity of what I had done, how could I choose to pursue my happiness? In reality, I made the present moment horrible to justify my obsession with and feelings about the past. I needed the present to be unlivable to support the general terribleness of my life leading up to it.

Even when I had the clarity to understand that I had to go forward for my family, I failed because I had not fully decided to live. I was stuck on existential matters played out in the past. I did not choose to pursue happiness. A sense of guilt and recognition of unfulfilled obligations is not the same thing as choosing to pursue individual happiness. I was going to inpatient and outpatient programs, but I was not moving forward toward anything, and I did not want to go anywhere or do anything. I was not trying to change myself. I was attending, but, like all else, doing so in a waking dream. It was not my life. I did not have a goal, and I was not moving toward one. I had not yet chosen to pursue happiness.

Feeling obliged to live and work is not the same thing as choosing to pursue happiness. Work will be required to achieve some form of happiness, but choosing to pursue happiness is not work. It is a choice. Without that personal conviction, the work I was doing to improve my lot was generally misdirected, guided by negative traits and impulses. Instead of really seeking to improve my situation, therapists and psychiatrists were my audience. Often, the personal interest of therapists is prurient and voyeuristic. I told stories that grew from truth but followed a path shaped by my general desire to have a story of origin like a comic-book hero. They loved learning about what dommes do, how a BDSM family and professional dungeon operate, the formal language, positions, and protocol of dominance and submission, how a TENS unit or sounds may be used, and on and on. Talking about my alternative life and intense devotions made me feel oh so edgy and cool. I felt extra super interesting and complex enough to have earned my problems. The therapists got super juicy and complex stories, enough symbiosis to fill any program or hospital stay. I could entertain without coming within a thousand fathoms of any real problem.

If I was bored, which was much of the time, and if I resented my caregivers, which was much of the time, I could be difficult. I was a skillful lawyer and an adept law professor with time on my hands. It did not take much to engage many of my keepers in a Socratic dialogue that would take them wherever I wanted to take them. Given that I was doing this because I was an obstreperous anus, the places I took them were forced admissions that what they were saying does not make sense, that they really did not know enough about the topic to be speaking, that really the opposite of what they said is correct. Mean. Pointless. Puerile. Wasteful. Counterproductive. Evasive. Egotistical. It looked like I was doing what I was supposed to be doing in whatever program, but whatever my life was, wherever it would be, I would remain a creature of whatever bucket of biases and fears I was at the moment. Even therapy to improve myself would be a playground for the things about me I should be seeking to correct.

A Socratic dialogue with a law professor is a tragedy akin to the tragedy Hemingway saw in every bullfight. In the end, the bull always dies. In the end, the student always loses. The success of the student, like that of the bull, can be measured only in how long he remains in the fight. The ill-fated bull gets to show his courage in the face of death. The matador merely murders with panache. The matador flaunts his mastery over an inferior and wounded victim like a law prof strutting up the aisle of the lecture hall while he tears down a student, but there is no "fight." Unfair. Pointless. Bloody. Fatal. When encountering the discomfort of my own problems and people who might help me, I chose to be the matador in my life drama. It would be facile to say that I was being uncooperative or even a jerk. I was far worse than that and knowingly so. I was holding on to something that turned those who might help change my lot into enemies. I used those pretended enemies as vehicles to rebuild a crumbled identity that was never more than a facade to begin with. The cycles of rebuilding and destruction were numerous and rapid. Much of the time I was the last, lone settler atop the tell formed by all my prior identities, dreaming of rebuilding the grand city that must have been there in antiquity. There never was a grand city, and I knew this. I also knew the dream itself was conjured to evade that truth.

The show on the ceiling ended because I encountered a therapist who would not play my games and insisted that I address present reality. You are turning forty? Unhappy with your career choices? Yawn. Manic sexual activity and intense attachments? Totally uninteresting. Committed Dominant/submissive relationship? Kink? Wake me up when you are done talking. But the emotions are so intense? Sure, "being in love is a bitch." You really should have figured this out in your teens. All these things are very real, but typical, nothing that should be an identity, nothing interesting, however intense and juicy the scene.

I am intense and creative. I had built ornate castles with mazes of walls and nested internal chambers that made for great site-seeing and difficult entry, but that is all it was. This guy was not going to be my voyeur or victim. I liked him. I respected him. I did not like my stories either and understood that while true, my stories were misdirections. Let's deal with career and disappointment later. Depression and suicide, that's the thing. That's the problem. That's what we need to figure out. Absolutely.

Perhaps in our third meeting, I was going off about *Woe is me, my family will be better off without me, I'm a coward for not doing what needs to be done*, you can fill in the rest. This guy stopped me and effectively called bullshit. He said, "You are a smart guy. What do you think happens to kids whose dad commits suicide when they are ages three and five?" He would not accept my internal life wrapped in poor assumptions, misapprehension, and the twisted logic of the crazy man. I tried to explain how different I am and how this is not the usual . . . He demanded a conversation about real things, not the nonsensical delusions that underlay my suicidal ideation.

He repeated, "What actually happens to those kids? Objectively, what happens?" Reality. Not how you feel or want things to be. What happens outside your fucked-up internal world? It is a terrible burden and pain to dump on toddlers. I would be gone, but they would never recover. What an unfair millstone to hang around a child's neck. They would have doubts about their own worth, anger, a very different life without a father, and on and on. I did not need to look at the stats. I knew what they would say. I did not need another punch. So I knew the move—get outside myself. How do my actions impact others I want to help? It's a strong move.

A life beyond the ceiling had to go forward because I was a father with young children who needed me. Reality. Inescapable. True. All the Hamlet business and rehashing of an overdose gone awry was fantasy. There was a present reality. I would have to live within it.

I go back to the moment with that therapist and that logic constantly. I have to live for my children. That is reality. There is a present reality in which I must live. Everything else is delusion powered by depression. My focus moves to the present, what is happening now, and what impact my present actions will have on the next moment. That is what I really have. That is where I really am.

Running took on new meaning and purpose in my life as a result. It was not diversion or part of a pursuit to change my body or grind it out of existence. It was what I was doing. It had all the virtues that have been spun out into this book—immediate, concrete, objective, measurable, healthful. I had goals and a path for my next steps. This made me happy and productive. Being a full-time dad was no longer a professional failure. It was a gift and a vocation for which I was suited and able to dedicate myself fully. Everything fell into place. I did not consciously choose to be happy, but I was doing things that had a profound impact on my life, that led to my productive growth and virtuous cycles of additional development, direction, and joy. I was a better person. I was a great dad and so very fortunate to make that my profession. The time with my children was precious, and I was aware of it at every step. I had seen other possible lives. The changes were thorough, profound, mental, physical. I am not the person who literally stared at a ceiling probably seven hours a day and slept an additional twelve hours for a decade. I do not want to go back to the table in the hospital.

The profundity of the changes and what I learned was possible pushed me into the philosophical quest that became this book.

My father gave me the concept and the words I did not have. The gift from my father was not just unraveling his assertion that happiness is a choice but giving me the concept and vocabulary to understand what underlay my path. Before I ended up breaking down during marathons and trying to understand how I ended up at the finish, I had made a choice to run. When I chose to run for the right reasons, to continue to improve and to do more than I thought possible and to find a way to do more on top of that, to move past pain and mortality to keep going, when I embarked on that path, I chose to be happy. And so I continue.

I wish I had fully understood and written this final section before I put a copy of this chapter in my father's casket. He gave me very few directives in life. It was not his style. He would offer his advice quietly and leave me to make the mistake against which he cautioned. He told me he wanted me to finish this. Perhaps he knew I would end up here.

Thank you, Dad.

EPILOGUE

Many Journeys, One Course

One of the best things about racing is seeing all the different people, sometimes people from all over the world. It's the only time I like talking to strangers. There are so many great stories, all my familiar friends—the soldiers and firefighters running in full kit for fallen comrades, the guy seemingly everywhere pushing a bed with his son with MS in it, the Sikh dude with knee-high tube socks dancing the entire 26.2 with a boom box on his shoulder. Even the common stories are fantastic—celebrating life after cancer, guys like me looking for meaning in the face of limitation and pain, at-risk kids in clubs, ex-convicts running with a judge working to save adult lives, ladies who started walking together five years ago and cannot believe they are at the starting line of a marathon, and, of course, dedicated runners at their glorious peak seeking a time. Everyone is nice to each other, high-fiving strangers, wishing them the best day of their lives. We have all been living our own paths, which range from the fit high-school runner doing it as a training exercise to those who will never walk again. We have all been seeking meaning and a way forward. All these paths from prisons and Afghanistan and Burbank and Peru and so, so, so many hospital beds, and they all lead to this moment, to the same time, to the same place. For that brief hour waiting, literally corralled together, many people know this. Our lives have come together, and we can celebrate each other's stories that we know intersect with ours in a meaningful way. We have different journeys to the start, but we will all cross the same finish line. For a moment, everyone recognizes that we share everything, our lives sharing one purpose and hope.

Then there is the starting gun, the high fives stop, and each runner begins his solitary trial. We allow our journeys to diverge. Many people will have the worst day of their life—pain and injury dashing dreams. Many people will have the best day of their life—ecstasy, victory, fun. Yet for everyone it remains the same start, the same course, and the same finish.

This is life.

ABOUT THE AUTHOR

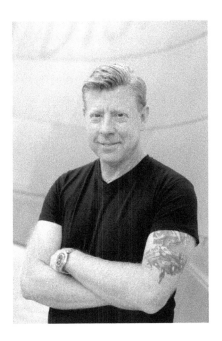

Craig Grossman is a retired lawyer and law professor and a former stay-at-home dad with degrees from Stanford University and Harvard Law School. A proud slow runner, Grossman has finished dozens of half marathons and five marathons, including, most recently, the 2023 New York City Marathon, his proudest (and slowest) result. A lover of Disneyland, Las Vegas, craft cocktails, the Los Angeles Philharmonic, and any costume event, he lives in Southern California with his family. *The Slow Runner's Nirvana* is his first book.

Milton Keynes UK
Ingram Content Group UK Ltd.
UKHW010839220224
438295UK00004B/231